Dear Future Exam Success Story:

Congratulations on your purchase of our study guide. Our goal in writing our study guide was to cover the content on the test, as well as provide insight into typical test taking mistakes and how to overcome them.

Standardized tests are a key component of being successful, which only increases the importance of doing well in the high-pressure high-stakes environment of test day. How well you do on this test will have a significant impact on your future- and we have the research and practical advice to help you execute on test day.

The product you're reading now is designed to exploit weaknesses in the test itself, and help you avoid the most common errors test takers frequently make.

How to use this study guide

We don't want to waste your time. Our study guide is fast-paced and fluff-free. We suggest going through it a number of times, as repetition is an important part of learning new information and concepts.

First, read through the study guide completely to get a feel for the content and organization. Read the general success strategies first, and then proceed to the content sections. Each tip has been carefully selected for its effectiveness.

Second, read through the study guide again, and take notes in the margins and highlight those sections where you may have a particular weakness.

Finally, bring the manual with you on test day and study it before the exam begins.

Your success is our success

We would be delighted to hear about your success. Send us an email and tell us your story. Thanks for your business and we wish you continued success-

Sincerely,

Mometrix Test Preparation Team

Need more help? Check out our flashcards at: http://MometrixFlashcards.com/HOBET

TABLE OF CONTENTS

Top 20 Test Taking Tips

1. Carefully follow all the test registration procedures
2. Know the test directions, duration, topics, question types, how many questions
3. Setup a flexible study schedule at least 3-4 weeks before test day
4. Study during the time of day you are most alert, relaxed, and stress free
5. Maximize your learning style; visual learner use visual study aids, auditory learner use auditory study aids
6. Focus on your weakest knowledge base
7. Find a study partner to review with and help clarify questions
8. Practice, practice, practice
9. Get a good night's sleep; don't try to cram the night before the test
10. Eat a well balanced meal
11. Know the exact physical location of the testing site; drive the route to the site prior to test day
12. Bring a set of ear plugs; the testing center could be noisy
13. Wear comfortable, loose fitting, layered clothing to the testing center; prepare for it to be either cold or hot during the test
14. Bring at least 2 current forms of ID to the testing center
15. Arrive to the test early; be prepared to wait and be patient
16. Eliminate the obviously wrong answer choices, then guess the first remaining choice
17. Pace yourself; don't rush, but keep working and move on if you get stuck
18. Maintain a positive attitude even if the test is going poorly
19. Keep your first answer unless you are positive it is wrong
20. Check your work, don't make a careless mistake

Reading

Paragraph and Passage Comprehension

Primary sources

When conducting research, it is important to depend on reputable primary sources. A primary source is the documentary evidence closest to the subject being studied. For instance, the primary sources for an essay about penguins would be photographs and recordings of the birds, as well as accounts of people who have studied penguins in person. A secondary source would be a review of a movie about penguins or a book outlining the observations made by others. A primary source should be credible and, if it is on a subject that is still being explored, recent. One way to assess the credibility of a work is to see how often it is mentioned in other books and articles on the same subject. Just by reading the works cited and bibliographies of other books, one can get a sense of what are the acknowledged authorities in the field.

Internet sources

The Internet was once considered a poor place to find sources for an essay or article, but its credibility has improved greatly over the years. Still, students need to exercise caution when performing research online. The best sources are those affiliated with established institutions, like universities, public libraries, and think tanks. Most newspapers are available online, and many of them allow the public to browse their archives. Magazines frequently offer similar services. When obtaining information from an unknown website, however, one must exercise considerably more caution. A website can be

considered trustworthy if it is referenced by other sites that are known to be reputable. Also, credible sites tend to be properly maintained and frequently updated. A site is easier to trust when the author provides some information about him or herself, including some credentials that indicate expertise in the subject matter.

Topic and summary sentences

Topic and summary sentences are a convenient way to encapsulate the main idea of a text. In some textbooks and academic articles, the author will place a topic or summary sentence at the beginning of each section as a means of preparing the reader for what is to come. Research suggests that the brain is more receptive to new information when it has been prepared by the presentation of the main idea or some key words. The phenomenon is somewhat akin to the primer coat of paint that allows subsequent coats of paint to absorb more easily. A good topic sentence will be clear and not contain any jargon. When topic or summary sentences are not provided, many good readers may jot down their own so that they can find their place in a text and refresh their memory.

Fact and opinion

Readers must always be conscious of the distinction between fact and opinion. A fact can be subjected to analysis and can be either proved or disproved. An opinion, on the other hand, is the author's personal feeling, which may not be alterable by research, evidence, or argument. If the author writes that the distance from New York to Boston is about two hundred miles, he is stating a fact. But if he writes that New York is too crowded, then he is giving an opinion, because there is no objective standard for overpopulation. An opinion may be indicated by words like *believe*, *think*, or

- 2 -

feel. Also, an opinion may be supported by facts: for instance, the author might give the population density of New York as a reason for why it is overcrowded. An opinion supported by fact tends to be more convincing. When authors support their opinions with other opinions, the reader is unlikely to be moved.

Biases and stereotypes

Every author has a point of view, but when an author ignores reasonable counterarguments or distorts opposing viewpoints, she is demonstrating a bias. A bias is evident whenever the author is unfair or inaccurate in his or her presentation. Bias may be intentional or unintentional, but it should always alert the reader to be skeptical of the argument being made. It should be noted that a biased author may still be correct. However, the author will be correct in spite of her bias, not because of it. A stereotype is like a bias, except that it is specifically applied to a group or place. Stereotyping is considered to be particularly abhorrent because it promotes negative generalizations about people. Many people are familiar with some of the hateful stereotypes of certain ethnic, religious, and cultural groups. Readers should be very wary of authors who stereotype. These faulty assumptions typically reveal the author's ignorance and lack of curiosity.

Identifying the logical conclusion

Identifying a logical conclusion is much like making an inference: it requires the reader to combine the information given by the text with what he already knows to make a supportable assertion. If a passage is written well, then the conclusion should be obvious even when it is unstated. If the author intends the reader to draw a certain conclusion, then all of his argumentation and detail should be leading toward it. One way to approach

the task of drawing conclusions is to make brief notes of all the points made by the author. When these are arranged on paper, they may clarify the logical conclusion. Another way to approach conclusions is to consider whether the reasoning of the author raises any pertinent questions. Sometimes it will be possible to draw several conclusions from a passage, and on occasion these will be conclusions that were never imagined by the author. It is essential, however, that these conclusions be supported directly by the text.

Topics and main ideas

One of the most important skills in reading comprehension is the identification of topics and main ideas. There is a subtle difference between these two features. The topic is the subject of a text, or what the text is about. The main idea, on the other hand, is the most important point being made by the author. The topic is usually expressed in a few words at the most, while the main idea often needs a full sentence to be completely defined. As an example, a short passage might have the topic of penguins and the main idea *Penguins are different from other birds in many ways*. In most nonfiction writing, the topic and the main idea will be stated directly, often in a sentence at the very beginning or end of the text. However, there are cases in which the reader must figure out an unstated topic or main idea. One way to approach this process is to read every sentence of the text, and try to come up with an overarching idea that is supported by each of those sentences.

Supporting details

Supporting details provide evidence and backing for the main point. All texts contain details, but they are only classified as supporting details when they serve to reinforce some larger point.

- 3 -

Supporting details are most commonly found in informative and persuasive texts. In some cases, they will be clearly indicated with words like *for example* or *for instance*, or they will be enumerated with words like *first*, *second*, and *last*. However, they may not be indicated with special words. As a reader, it is important to consider whether the author's supporting details really back up his or her main point. Supporting details can be factual and correct but still not relevant to the author's point. Conversely, supporting details can seem pertinent but be ineffective because they are based on opinion or assertions that cannot be proven.

Themes

Themes are seldom expressed directly in a text, so they can be difficult to identify. A theme is an issue, an idea, or a question raised by the text. For instance, a theme of William Shakespeare's *Hamlet* is indecision, as the title character explores his own psyche and the results of his failure to make bold choices. A great work of literature may have many themes, and the reader is justified in identifying any for which he or she can find support. One common characteristic of themes is that they raise more questions than they answer. In a good piece of fiction, the author is not always trying to convince the reader, but is instead trying to elevate the reader's perspective and encourage him to consider the themes more deeply. When reading, one can identify themes by constantly asking what general issues the text is addressing. A good way to evaluate an author's approach to a theme is to begin reading with a question in mind (for example, how does this text approach the theme of love?) and then look for evidence in the text that addresses that question.

Persuasive writing

In a persuasive essay, the author is attempting to change the reader's mind or convince him of something he did not believe previously. There are several identifying characteristics of persuasive writing. One is opinion presented as fact. When an author attempts to persuade the reader, he often presents his or her opinions as if they were fact. A reader must be on guard for statements that sound factual but which cannot be subjected to research, observation, or experiment. Another characteristic of persuasive writing is emotional language. An author will often try to play on the reader's emotion by appealing to his sympathy or sense of morality. When an author uses colorful or evocative language with the intent of arousing the reader's passions, it is likely that he is attempting to persuade. Finally, in many cases a persuasive text will give an unfair explanation of opposing positions, if these positions are mentioned at all.

Appeal to emotion

Sometimes, authors will appeal to the reader's emotion in an attempt to persuade or to distract the reader from the weakness of the argument. For instance, the author may try to inspire the pity of the reader by delivering a heart-rending story. An author also might use the bandwagon approach, in which he suggests that his opinion is correct because it is held by the majority. Some authors resort to name-calling, in which insults and harsh words are delivered to the opponent in an attempt to distract. In advertising, a common appeal is the testimonial, in which a famous person endorses a product. Of course, the fact that a celebrity likes something should not really mean anything to the reader. These and other emotional appeals are usually evidence of poor reasoning and a weak argument.

Logical fallacy

False analogy

A logical fallacy is a failure of reasoning. As a reader, it is important to recognize logical fallacies, because they diminish the value of the author's message. The four most common logical fallacies in writing are the false analogy, circular reasoning, false dichotomy, and overgeneralization. In a false analogy, the author suggests that two things are similar, when in fact they are different. This fallacy is often committed when the author is attempting to convince the reader that something unknown is like something relatively familiar. The author takes advantage of the reader's ignorance to make this false comparison. One example might be the following statement: *Failing to tip a waitress is like stealing money out of somebody's wallet*. Of course, failing to tip is very rude, especially when the service has been good, but people are not arrested for failing to tip as they would for stealing money from a wallet. To compare stingy diners with thieves is a false analogy.

Circular reasoning

Circular reasoning is one of the more difficult logical fallacies to identify, because it is typically hidden behind dense language and complicated sentences. Reasoning is described as circular when it offers no support for assertions other than restating them in different words. Put another way, a circular argument refers to itself as evidence of truth. A simple example of circular argument is when a person uses a word to define itself, such as saying *Niceness is the state of being nice*. If the reader does not know what *nice* means, then this definition will not be very useful. In a text, circular reasoning is usually more complex. For instance, an author might say *Poverty is a problem for society because it creates trouble for people throughout the community*. It is redundant to say that poverty is a problem because it creates trouble. When an author engages in circular reasoning, it is often because he or she has not fully thought out the argument, or cannot come up with any legitimate justifications.

False dichotomy

One of the most common logical fallacies is the false dichotomy, in which the author creates an artificial sense that there are only two possible alternatives in a situation. This fallacy is common when the author has an agenda and wants to give the impression that his view is the only sensible one. A false dichotomy has the effect of limiting the reader's options and imagination. An example of a false dichotomy is the statement *You need to go to the party with me, otherwise you'll just be bored at home*. The speaker suggests that the only other possibility besides being at the party is being bored at home. But this is not true, as it is perfectly possible to be entertained at home, or even to go somewhere other than the party. Readers should always be wary of the false dichotomy: when an author limits alternatives, it is always wise to ask whether he is being valid.

Overgeneralization

Overgeneralization is a logical fallacy in which the author makes a claim that is so broad it cannot be proved or disproved. In most cases, overgeneralization occurs when the author wants to create an illusion of authority, or when he is using sensational language to sway the opinion of the reader. For instance, in the sentence *Everybody knows that she is a terrible teacher*, the author makes an assumption that cannot really be believed. This kind of statement is made when the author wants to create the illusion of consensus when none actually exists: it may be that most people have a negative view of the teacher, but to say that *everybody* feels that way is an exaggeration. When a reader spots

- 5 -

overgeneralization, she should become skeptical about the argument that is being made, because an author will often try to hide a weak or unsupported assertion behind authoritative language.

Informative texts

An informative text is written to educate and enlighten the reader. Informative texts are almost always nonfiction, and are rarely structured as a story. The intention of an informative text is to deliver information in the most comprehensible way possible, so the structure of the text is likely to be very clear. In an informative text, the thesis statement is often in the first sentence. The author may use some colorful language, but is likely to put more emphasis on clarity and precision. Informative essays do not typically appeal to the emotions. They often contain facts and figures, and rarely include the opinion of the author. Sometimes a persuasive essay can resemble an informative essay, especially if the author maintains an even tone and presents his or her views as if they were established fact.

Entertaining texts

The success or failure of an author's intent to entertain is determined by those who read the author's work. Entertaining texts may be either fiction or nonfiction, and they may describe real or imagined people, places, and events. Entertaining texts are often narratives, or stories. A text that is written to entertain is likely to contain colorful language that engages the imagination and the emotions. Such writing often features a great deal of figurative language, which typically enlivens its subject matter with images and analogies. Though an entertaining text is not usually written to persuade or inform, it may accomplish both of these tasks. An entertaining text may appeal to

the reader's emotions and cause him or her to think differently about a particular subject. In any case, entertaining texts tend to showcase the personality of the author more so than do other types of writing.

Expression of feelings

When an author intends to express feelings, she may use colorful and evocative language. An author may write emotionally for any number of reasons. Sometimes, the author will do so because she is describing a personal situation of great pain or happiness. Sometimes an author is attempting to persuade the reader, and so will use emotion to stir up the passions. It can be easy to identify this kind of expression when the writer uses phrases like *I felt* and *I sense*. However, sometimes the author will simply describe feelings without introducing them. As a reader, it is important to recognize when an author is expressing emotion, and not to become overwhelmed by sympathy or passion. A reader should maintain some detachment so that he or she can still evaluate the strength of the author's argument or the quality of the writing.

Predictions based on prior knowledge

A prediction is a guess about what will happen next. Readers are constantly making predictions based on what they have read and what they already know. Making predictions is an important part of being an active reader. Consider the following sentence: *Staring at the computer screen in shock, Kim blindly reached over for the brimming glass of water on the shelf to her side.* The sentence suggests that Kim is agitated and that she is not looking at the glass she is going to pick up, so a reader might predict that she is going to knock the glass over. Of course, not every prediction will be accurate: perhaps Kim will pick the glass up cleanly. Nevertheless, the author has certainly created the expectation that the water might be spilled. Predictions are always subject to revision as the reader acquires more information.

Making inferences

A text often makes claims and suggests ideas without stating them directly. An inference is a piece of information that is implied but not written outright by the author. For instance, consider the following sentence: *Mark made more money that week than he had in the previous year.* From this sentence, the reader can infer that Mark either has not made much money in the previous year or made a great deal of money that week. Often, a reader can use information he or she already knows to make inferences. Take as an example the sentence *When his coffee arrived, he looked around the table for the silver cup.* Many people know that cream is typically served in a silver cup, so using their own base of knowledge they can infer that the subject of this sentence takes his coffee with cream. Making inferences requires concentration, attention, and practice.

Problem-solution text structure

Some nonfiction texts are organized to present a problem followed by a solution. In this type of text, it is common for the problem to be explained before the solution is offered. In some cases, as when the problem is well known, the solution may be briefly introduced at the beginning. Other times, the entire passage will focus on the solution, and the problem will be referenced only occasionally. This is common when the author can assume that the reading audience is already familiar with the problem. Some texts will outline multiple solutions to a problem, leaving the reader to choose among them. If the author has an interest or an allegiance to one

solution, he may fail to mention or may describe inaccurately some of the other solutions. Readers should be careful of the author's agenda when reading a problem-solution text. Only by understanding the author's point of view and interests can one develop a proper judgment of the proposed solution.

Descriptive text

In a sense, almost all writing is descriptive, insofar as it seeks to describe events, ideas, or people to the reader. Some texts, however, are primarily concerned with description. A descriptive text focuses on a particular subject, and attempts to depict it in a way that will be clear to the reader. Descriptive texts contain many adjectives and adverbs, words that give shades of meaning and create a more detailed mental picture for the reader. A descriptive text fails when it is unclear or vague to the reader. On the other hand, however, a descriptive text that compiles too much detail can be boring and overwhelming to the reader. A descriptive text will certainly be informative, and it may be persuasive and entertaining as well. Descriptive writing is a challenge for the author, but when it is done well, it can be fun to read.

Sequence

A reader must be able to identify a text's sequence, or the order in which things happen. Often, and especially when the sequence is very important to the author, it is indicated with signal words like *first*, *then*, *next*, and *last*. However, sometimes a sequence is merely implied and must be noted by the reader. Consider the sentence *He walked in the front door and switched on the hall lamp.* Clearly, the man did not turn the lamp on before he walked in the door, so the implied sequence is that he first walked in the door and then turned on the lamp. Texts do not always proceed in an orderly sequence from first to last: sometimes, they begin at the end and then start over at the beginning. As a reader, it can be useful to make brief notes to clarify the sequence.

Comparison and contrast

When an author describes the ways in which two things are alike, he or she is comparing them. When the author describes the ways in which two things are different, he or she is contrasting them. The "compare and contrast" essay is one of the most common forms in nonfiction. It is often signaled with certain words: a comparison may be indicated with such words as *both, same, like, too,* and *as well;* while a contrast may be indicated by words like *but, however, on the other hand, instead,* and *yet.* Of course, comparisons and contrasts may be implicit without using any such signaling language. A single sentence may both compare and contrast. Consider the sentence *Brian and Sheila love ice cream, but Brian prefers vanilla and Sheila prefers strawberry.* In one sentence, the author has described both a similarity (love of ice cream) and a difference (favorite flavor).

Cause and effect

One of the most common text structures is cause and effect. A cause is an act or event that makes something happen, and an effect is the thing that happens as a result of that cause. A cause-and-effect relationship is not always explicit, but there are some words in English that signal causality, such as *since, because,* and *as a result.* As an example, consider the sentence *Because the sky was clear, Ron did not bring an umbrella.* The cause is the clear sky, and the effect is that Ron did not bring an umbrella. However, sometimes the cause-and-effect relationship will not be clearly noted. For instance, the sentence *He was late and missed the meeting* does not contain any signaling words, but it still contains a cause (he was late) and an effect (he missed the meeting). It is possible for a single cause to have multiple effects, or for a single effect to have multiple causes. Also, an effect can in turn be the cause of another effect, in what is known as a cause-and-effect chain.

Identifying an author's position

In order to be an effective reader, one must pay attention to the author's position and purpose. Even those texts that seem objective and impartial, like textbooks, have some sort of position and bias. Readers need to take these positions into account when considering the author's message. When an author uses emotional language or clearly favors one side of an argument, his position is clear. However, the author's position may be evident not only in what he writes, but in what he doesn't write. For this reason, it is sometimes necessary to review some other texts on the same topic in order to develop a view of the author's position. If this is not possible, then it may be useful to acquire a little background personal information about the author. When the only source of information is the text, however, the reader should look for language and argumentation that seems to indicate a particular stance on the subject.

Purpose

Identifying the purpose of an author is usually easier than identifying her position. In most cases, the author has no interest in hiding his or her purpose. A text that is meant to entertain, for instance, should be obviously written to please the reader. Most narratives, or stories, are written to entertain, though they may also inform or persuade. Informative texts are easy to identify as well. The most difficult purpose of a text to identify is persuasion, because the author has an interest in making this purpose hard to detect. When a person knows that the author is trying to convince him, he is automatically more wary and skeptical of the argument. For this reason persuasive texts often try to establish an entertaining tone, hoping to amuse the reader into agreement, or an informative tone, hoping to create an appearance of authority and objectivity.

An author's purpose is often evident in the organization of the text. For instance, if the text has headings and subheadings, if key terms are in bold, and if the author makes his main idea clear from the beginning, then the likely purpose of the text is to inform. If the author begins by making a claim and then makes various arguments to support that claim, the purpose is probably to persuade. If the author is telling a story, or is more interested in holding the attention of the reader than in making a particular point or delivering information, then his purpose is most likely to entertain. As a reader, it is best to judge an author on how well he accomplishes his purpose. In other words, it is not entirely fair to complain that a textbook is boring: if the text is clear and easy to understand, then the author has done his job. Similarly, a storyteller should not be judged too harshly for getting some facts wrong, so long as he is able to give pleasure to the reader.

Narrative passage

A narrative passage is a story. Narratives can be fiction or nonfiction. However, there are a few elements that a text must have in order to be classified as a narrative. To begin with, the text must have a plot. That is, it must describe a series of events. If it is a good narrative, these events will be interesting and emotionally engaging to the reader. A narrative also has characters. These could be people, animals, or even inanimate objects, so long as they participate in the plot. A narrative passage often contains figurative language, which is meant to stimulate the imagination of the reader by making comparisons and observations. A metaphor, which is a description of one thing in terms of another, is a common piece of figurative language. *The moon was a frosty snowball* is an example of a metaphor: it is obviously untrue in the literal sense, but it suggests a certain mood for the reader. Narratives often proceed in a clear sequence, but they do not need to do so.

Expository passage

An expository passage aims to inform and enlighten the reader. It is nonfiction and usually centers around a simple, easily defined topic. Since the goal of exposition is to teach, such a passage should be as clear as possible. It is common for an expository passage to contain helpful organizing words, like *first*, *next*, *for example*, and *therefore*. These words keep the reader oriented in the text. Although expository passages do not need to feature colorful language and artful writing, they are often more effective when they do. For a reader, the challenge of expository passages is to maintain steady attention. Expository passages are not always about subjects in which a reader will naturally be interested, and the writer is often more concerned with clarity and comprehensibility than with engaging the reader. For this reason, many expository passages are dull. Making notes is a good way to maintain focus when reading an expository passage.

Technical passage

A technical passage is written to describe a complex object or process. Technical writing is common in medical and technological fields, in which complicated mathematical, scientific, and engineering ideas need to be explained simply and clearly. To ease comprehension, a technical passage usually proceeds in a very logical order. Technical passages often have clear headings and subheadings, which are used to keep the reader oriented in the text. It is also common for these passages to break sections up with numbers or letters. Many technical passages look more like an outline than a piece of prose. The amount of jargon or difficult vocabulary will vary in a technical passage depending on the intended audience. As much as possible, technical passages try to avoid language that the reader will have to research in order to understand the message. Of course, it is not always possible to avoid jargon.

Persuasive passage

A persuasive passage is meant to change the reader's mind or lead her into agreement with the author. The persuasive intent may be obvious, or it may be quite difficult to discern. In some cases, a persuasive passage will be indistinguishable from an informative passage: it will make an assertion and offer supporting details. However, a persuasive passage is more likely to make claims based on opinion and to appeal to the reader's emotions. Persuasive passages may not describe alternate positions and, when they do, they often display significant bias. It may be clear that a persuasive passage is giving the author's viewpoint, or the passage may adopt a seemingly objective tone. A persuasive passage is successful if it can make a convincing argument and win the trust of the reader.

Historical context

Historical context has a profound influence on literature: the events, knowledge base, and assumptions of an author's time color every aspect of his or her work. Sometimes, authors hold opinions and use language that would be considered inappropriate or immoral in a modern setting, but that was acceptable in the author's time. As a reader, one should consider how the historical context influenced a work and also how today's opinions and ideas shape the way modern readers read the works of the past. For instance, in most societies of the past, women were treated as second-class citizens. An author who wrote in 18th-century England might sound sexist to modern readers, even if that author was relatively feminist in his time. Readers should not have to excuse the faulty assumptions and prejudices of the past, but they should appreciate that a person's thoughts and words are, in part, a result of the time and culture in which they live or lived, and it is perhaps unfair to expect writers to avoid all of the errors of their times.

Similar themes across cultures

Even a brief study of world literature suggests that writers from vastly different cultures address similar themes. For instance, works like the *Odyssey* and *Hamlet* both tackle the individual's battle for self-control and independence. In every culture, authors address themes of personal growth and the struggle for maturity. Another universal theme is the conflict between the individual and society. In works as culturally disparate as *Native Son*, the *Aeneid*, and *1984*, authors dramatize how people struggle to maintain their personalities and dignity in large, sometimes oppressive groups. Finally, many cultures have versions of the hero's (or heroine's) journey, in which an adventurous person must overcome many obstacles in order to gain greater knowledge, power, and perspective. Some famous works that treat this theme are the *Epic of Gilgamesh*, Dante's *Divine Comedy*, and *Don Quixote.*

Difference in addressing themes in various cultures and genres

Authors from different genres (for instance poetry, drama, novel, short story) and cultures may address similar themes, but they often do so quite differently. For instance, poets are likely to address subject matter obliquely, through the use of images and allusions. In a play, on the other hand, the author is more likely to dramatize themes by using characters to express opposing viewpoints. This disparity is known as a dialectical approach. In a novel, the author does not need to express themes directly; rather, they can be illustrated through events and actions. In some regional literatures, like those of Greece or England, authors use more irony: their works have characters that express views and make decisions that are clearly disapproved of by the author. In Latin America, there is a great tradition of using supernatural events to illustrate themes about real life. In China and Japan, authors frequently use well-established regional forms (haiku, for instance) to organize their treatment of universal themes.

Informational Source Comprehension

Following directions

Technical passages often require the reader to follow a set of directions. For many people, especially those who are tactile or visual learners, this can be a difficult process. It is important to approach a set of directions differently than other texts. First of all, it is a good idea to scan the directions to determine whether special equipment or preparations are needed. Sometimes in a recipe, for instance, the author fails to mention that the oven should be preheated first, and then halfway through the process, the cook is supposed to be baking. After briefly reading the directions, the reader should return to the first step. When following directions, it is appropriate to complete each step before moving on to the next. If this is not possible, it is useful at least to visualize each step before reading the next.

Word meaning from context

One of the benefits of reading is the expansion of the vocabulary. In order to obtain this benefit, however, one needs to know how to identify the definition of a word from its context. This means defining a word based on the words around it and the way it is used in a sentence. For instance, consider the following sentence: *The elderly scholar spent his evenings hunched over arcane texts that few other people even knew existed.* The adjective *arcane* is uncommon, but the reader can obtain significant information about it based on its use here. Based on the fact that few other people know of their existence, the reader can assume that arcane texts must be rare and only of interest to a few people. And, because they are being read by an elderly scholar, the reader can assume that they focus on difficult academic subjects. Sometimes, words can even be defined by what they are not. For instance, consider the following sentence: *Ron's fealty to his parents was not shared by Karen, who disobeyed their every command.* Because someone who disobeys is not demonstrating *fealty*, the word can be inferred to mean something like obedience or respect.

Dictionary entry

Many words can be defined by their context, but in other situations it will be necessary to read the word's definition in a dictionary. Dictionary entries are in alphabetical order. Many words have more than one definition, in which case the definitions will be numbered. Also, if a word can be used as different parts of speech, its various definitions in those different capacities may be separated. A sample entry might look like this:

WELL: (adverb) 1. in a good way (noun) 1. a hole drilled into the earth
The correct definition of a word will vary depending on how it is used in a sentence. When looking up a word found while reading, the best way to determine the relevant definition is to substitute the dictionary's definitions for the word in the text, and select the definition that seems most appropriate.

Food and medicine labels

The Food and Drug Administration has strict mandates for the information that must be included on food and medicine labels. For instance, a food label must list the corresponding food's number of calories, total fat, cholesterol, sodium, protein, and carbohydrates, among others. Also, a food label will usually contain a list of the vitamins that can be found in the product. Most importantly, a food label lists the serving size, which is the portion of the product for which the vitamin and nutrient values are true. Some food manufacturers use odd serving sizes to make it look as if a product is healthier than it is. When making a comparison, one should always calculate the amount of nutrients per unit of measure (grams or fluid ounces, for example) to account for these serving size distortions.

Medicine labels contain a wealth of information that can be used to make comparisons and informed purchases. Every medicine label must have detailed and comprehensive instructions regarding dosage, including how much and how often the medicine should be taken. A label will also include warning

information, and what to do in case of overdose or adverse reaction. Medicine labels will have a complete list of ingredients, but will isolate the active ingredients, which are those that accomplish the advertised purpose of the product. Often, generic versions of a medicine have the same active ingredients as more expensive name-brand versions. Finally, a label will specify when a medication should not be taken by certain people, like the elderly or pregnant women. When comparing medicines, it is important to isolate the most crucial information: dosage schedule, active ingredients, and counter-indications.

Information from printed communication

<u>Memo</u>
A memo (short for *memorandum*) is a common form of written communication. There is a standard format for these documents. It is typical for there to be a heading at the top indicating the author, date, and recipient. In some cases, this heading will also include the author's title and the name of his or her institution. Below this information will be the body of the memo. These documents are typically written by and for members of the same organization. They usually contain a plan of action, a request for information on a specific topic, or a response to such a request. Memos are considered to be official documents, and so are usually written in a formal style. Many memos are organized with numbers or bullet points, which make it easier for the reader to identify key ideas.

<u>Posted announcement</u>
People post announcements for all sorts of occasions. Many people are familiar with notices for lost pets, yard sales, and landscaping services. In order to be effective, these announcements need to contain all of the information the reader

requires to act on the message. For instance, a lost pet announcement needs to include a good description of the animal and a contact number for the owner. A yard sale notice should include the address, date, and hours of the sale, as well as a brief description of the products that will be available there. When composing an announcement, it is important to consider the perspective of the audience: what will they need to know in order to respond to the message? Although a posted announcement should try to use color and decoration to attract the eye of the passerby, it must also convey the necessary information.

Classified advertisement

Classified advertisements, or *ads*, are used to sell or buy goods, to attract business, to make romantic connections, and to do countless other things. They are an inexpensive, and sometimes free, way to make a brief pitch. Classified ads used to be found only in newspapers or special advertising circulars, but there are now many famous online listings as well. The style of these ads has remained basically the same. An ad usually begins with a word or phrase indicating what is being sold or sought. Then, the listing will give a brief description of the product or service. Because space is limited and costly in newspapers, classified ads there will often contain abbreviations for common attributes. For instance, two common abbreviations are *bk* for *black*, and *obo* for *or best offer*. Classified ads will then usually conclude by listing the price (or the amount the seeker is willing to pay), followed by contact information like a telephone number or email address.

Index

A nonfiction book will typically have an index at the end so that the reader can easily find information about particular topics. An index lists the topics in alphabetical order. The names of people are listed with the last name first. For example, *Adams, John* would come before *Washington, George*. To the right of the entry, the relevant page numbers are listed. When a topic is mentioned over several pages, the index will often connect these pages with a dash. For instance, if the subject is mentioned from pages 35 to 42 and again on 53, then the index entry will be labeled as *35-42, 53*. Some entries will have subsets, which are listed below the main entry, indented slightly, and placed in alphabetical order. This is common for subjects that are discussed frequently in the book. For instance, in a book about Elizabethan drama, William Shakespeare will likely be an important topic. Beneath Shakespeare's name in the index, there might be listings for *death of*, *dramatic works of*, *life of*, etc. These more specific entries help the reader refine his search.

Table of contents

Most books, magazines, and journals have a table of contents at the beginning. This helps the reader find the different parts of the book. The table of contents is usually found a page or two after the title page in a book, and on the first few pages of a magazine. However, many magazines now place the table of contents in the midst of an overabundance of advertisements, because they know readers will have to look at the ads as they search for the table. The standard orientation for a table of contents is the sections of the book listed along the left side, with the initial page number for each along the right. It is common in a book for the prefatory material (preface, introduction, etc.) to be numbered with Roman numerals. The contents are always listed in order from the beginning of the book to the end.

Road atlas

A student must be able to find information in various sources. A road atlas is a collection of maps specially designed for drivers. It is useful for finding the distances between places, the correct roads and highways for reaching a given destination, and the relative positions of places in a certain geographic area. Most road atlases have a table at the beginning that illustrates the distance in miles between any two major cities. These tables are set up like a grid, with cities listed along the left and top sides. To find the distance between two places, follow the row of the first place perpendicular from the left until it intersects with the column of the second place. Some atlases have similar tables indicating the estimated travel time from one location to another.

Card catalog

Although card catalogs are rarely seen in the physical world anymore, they still exist in most libraries in an online, digital format. These catalogs contain a wealth of information about the contents of the library. A typical card catalog entry contains the title, name of the author, year of publication, publisher, number of pages, and reference number in the Library of Congress. Most importantly, perhaps, card catalogs contain a brief summary of the book, so that a potential reader or researcher can get an idea of its contents. Many online card catalogs allow easy navigation to books on the same subject, by the same author, or close by on the library shelves. In any case, the card catalog entry will contain the library call number so that the researcher can find the book.

Dictionary

Dictionaries contain information about words. The words in a dictionary are listed in alphabetical order. A standard dictionary entry begins with a pronunciation guide for the word. The entry will also give the word's part of speech: that is, whether it is a noun, verb, adjective, etc. Some words can serve multiple functions in a sentence. For instance, the word *tough* is both an adjective meaning coarse or durable and a noun referring to a thug or a ruffian. The main component of a dictionary entry is the list of definitions. Some words have dozens of definitions. A good dictionary will also include the word's origins, including the language from which it is derived and its meaning in that language. This information is known as the word's etymology.

Owner's manual

An owner's manual is the appropriate source of information for a purchased product. An owner's manual is mainly devoted to the operation and maintenance of the product. It will often begin with a brief outline of the product's parts and method of operation. Most manuals will contain the products specifications: that is, the precise details about its components and features. For the most part, though, the owner's manual will be devoted to the routine repairs and care that a non-expert owner can be expected to provide. In the owner's manual for a car, for instance, there will be instructions for tasks like changing the oil, replacing windshield wipers, and presetting stations on the radio. An owner's manual is unlikely to contain instructions for complex repairs that require special equipment. Finally, the owner's manual will often detail the service warranty associated with the product.

Database information

Databases are systems for storing and organizing large amounts of information.

As personal computers have become more common and accessible, databases have become ever more present. The standard layout of a database is as a grid, with labels along the left side and the top. The horizontal rows and vertical columns that make up the grid are usually numbered or lettered, so that a particular square within the database might have a name like A3 or G5. Databases are good for storing information that can be expressed succinctly. They are most commonly used to store numerical data, but they also can be used to store the answers to yes-no questions and other brief data points. Information that is ambiguous (that is, has multiple possible meanings) or difficult to express in a few words is not appropriate for a database.

Encyclopedia

Encyclopedias used to be the best source for general information on a range of common subjects. Many people took pride in owning a set of encyclopedias, which were often written by top researchers. Now, encyclopedias largely exist online. Although they no longer have a preeminent place in general scholarship, these digital encyclopedias now often feature audio and video clips. A good encyclopedia remains the best place to obtain basic information about a well-known topic. There are also specialty encyclopedias that cover more obscure or expert information. For instance, there are many medical encyclopedias that contain the detail and sophistication required by doctors. For a regular person researching a subject like ostriches, Pennsylvania, or the Crimean War, an encyclopedia is a good source.

Headings and subheadings

Many informative texts, especially textbooks, use headings and subheadings for organization. Headings and subheadings are typically printed in larger and bolder fonts, and are often in a different color than the main body of the text. Headings may be larger than subheadings. Also, headings and subheadings are not always complete sentences. A heading announces the topic that will be addressed in the text below. Headings are meant to alert the reader to what is about to come. Subheadings announce the topics of smaller sections within the entire section indicated by the heading. So, for instance, the heading of a section in a science textbook might be *AMPHIBIANS*, and within that section might be subheadings for *Frogs*, *Salamanders*, and *Newts*. Readers should always pay close attention to headings and subheadings, because they prime the brain for the information that is about to be delivered, and because they make it easy to go back and find particular details in a long text.

Bold text and underlining

Authors will often incorporate text features like bold text, italics, and underlining to communicate meaning to the reader. When text is made bold, it is often because the author wants to emphasize the point that is being made. Bold text indicates importance. Also, many textbooks place key terms in bold. This not only draws the reader's attention, but also makes it easy to find these terms when reviewing before a test. Underlining serves a similar purpose. It is often used to suggest emphasis. However, underlining is also used on occasion beneath the titles of books, magazines, and works of art. This was more common when people used typewriters, on which italics are not possible. Now that word processor software is more prevalent, italics are generally used for longer works.

Italics

Italics, like bold text and underlines, are used to emphasize important words, phrases, and sentences in a text. However, italics have other uses as well. A word is placed in italics when it is being discussed as a word: that is, when it is being defined or its use in a sentence is being described. For instance, it is appropriate to use italics when saying that *esoteric* is an unusual adjective. Italics are also used for long or large works, like books, magazines, long operas, and epic poems. Shorter works are typically placed within quotation marks. A reader should note how an author uses italics, as this is a marker of style and tone. Some authors use them frequently, creating a tone of high emotion, while others are more restrained in their use, suggesting calm and reason.

Line graph

A line graph is typically used for measuring trends over time. It is set up along a vertical and a horizontal axis. The variables being measured are listed along the left side and the bottom side of the axes. Points are then plotted along the graph, such that they correspond with their values for each variable. For instance, imagine a line graph measuring a person's income for each month of the year. If the person earned $1500 in January, there would be a point directly above January, perpendicular to the horizontal axis, and directly to the right of $1500, perpendicular to the vertical axis. Once all of the lines are plotted, they are connected with a line from left to right. This line provides a nice visual illustration of the general trends. For instance, using the earlier example, if the line sloped up, it would be clear that the person's income had increased over the course of the year.

Bar graph

The bar graph is one of the most common visual representations of information. Bar graphs are used to illustrate sets of numerical data. The graph has a vertical axis, along which numbers are listed, and a horizontal axis, along which categories, words, or some other indicators are placed. One example of a bar graph is a depiction of the respective heights of famous basketball players: the vertical axis would contain numbers ranging from five to eight feet, and the horizontal axis would contain the names of the players. The length of the bar above the player's name would illustrate his height, as the top of the bar would stop perpendicular to the height listed along the left side. In this representation, then, it would be easy to see that Yao Ming is taller than Michael Jordan, because Yao's bar would be higher.

Pie chart

A pie chart, also known as a circle graph, is useful for depicting how a single unit or category is divided. The standard pie chart is a circle within which wedges have been cut and labeled. Each of these wedges is proportional in size to its part of the whole. For instance, consider a pie chart representing a student's budget. If the student spends half her money on rent, then the pie chart will represent that amount with a line through the center of the pie. If she spends a quarter of her money on food, there will be a line extending from the edge of the circle to the center at a right angle to the line depicting rent. This illustration would make it clear that the student spends twice as much money on rent as she does on food. The pie chart is only appropriate for showing how a whole is divided.

Scale readings of standard measurement instruments

The scales used on standard measurement instruments are fairly easy to read with a little practice. Take the ruler as an example. A typical ruler has different units along each long edge. One side measures inches, and the other measures centimeters. The units are specified close to the zero reading for the ruler. Note that the ruler does not begin measuring from its outermost edge. The zero reading is a black line a tiny distance inside of the edge. On the inches side, each inch is indicated with a long black line and a number. Each half-inch is noted with a slightly shorter line. Quarter-inches are noted with still shorter lines, eighth-inches are noted with even shorter lines, and sixteenth of an inch are noted with the shortest lines of all. On the centimeter side, the second-largest black lines indicate half-centimeters, and the smaller lines indicate tenths of centimeters, otherwise known as millimeters.

Legend or key of a map

Almost all maps contain a key, or legend, that defines the symbols used on the map for various landmarks. This key is usually placed in a corner of the map. It should contain listings for all of the important symbols on the map. Of course, these symbols will vary depending on the nature of the map. A road map uses different colored lines to indicate roads, highways, and interstates. A legend might also indicate the different dots and squares that are used to indicate towns of various sizes. The legend may contain information about the map's scale, though this may be elsewhere on the map. Many legends will contain special symbols, such as a picnic table indicating a campground.

Calculating the most economical buy

When deciding between similar products, it can be difficult to discern the most economical choice. Before making a final decision, one should evaluate the itemized price of each product. That is, one should break down the price into its components: base cost, tax, and delivery charges, if any. When purchasing a product that is sold in different amounts (like cereal or shampoo), one should calculate and compare price per unit. As an example, imagine one set of blank CDs costs $15 for 10, while another costs $20 for 12. The per-unit cost can be calculated by dividing the total cost by the number of units: $15/10 = 1.5$ and $20/12 =$ about 1.67, so the first set of CDs costs $1.50 per disc and the second costs approximately $1.67 per disc. By this measure, the pack of 10 is the more economical choice.

Yellow Pages

The Yellow Pages of the phone book contain commercial listings for businesses that provide services to the general public. The listings are organized according to the type of service being offered: there are sections for florists, auto mechanics, and pizza restaurants. These categories are placed in alphabetical order, and within each category, the listings are in alphabetical order. A basic listing in the yellow pages will include the name of the business, the address, and the phone number. However, some merchants elect to pay extra and have large advertisements alongside their listing in the yellow pages. For instance, a restaurant might buy enough space to print their entire menu.

Items and costs

Reading a table, as for instance a menu or a set of movie listings, takes practice. In a typical menu format, the price is listed directly across from the item. However, in some cases all of the items in a category (desserts, for example) have the same price, and this price is given at the top of the section. Sometimes, the prices of additives (like 75 cents for cheese on a hamburger) are listed at the bottom of the section. In some restaurants, prices are listed without the dollar sign ($). Also, some restaurants automatically subtract a certain amount of money for the server's tip, and this information is usually listed at the bottom of the menu page. On a set of movie listings, it is typical for the times at which a picture is showing to be listed in chronological order, as in the following example: *Harold Goes to Mars – 1:15, 3:30, 5:45, 8, 10:30*. Note that times that are exactly on the hour do not include minutes. Also, in some places a period is used instead of a colon to separate hours and minutes.

Mathematics

Numbers and Operations

Converting percents, fractions, and decimals

Example 1

15% can be written as a fraction and as a decimal. 15% written as a fraction is $\frac{15}{100}$ which equals $\frac{3}{20}$. 15% written as a decimal is 0.15.

To convert a percent to a fraction, follow these steps:

1) Write the percent over 100 because percent means "per one hundred." So, 15% can be written as $\frac{15}{100}$.

2) Fractions should be written in simplest form, which means that the numbers in the numerator and denominator should be reduced if possible. Both 15 and 100 can be divided by 5.

3) Therefore, $\frac{15 \div 5}{100 \div 5} = \frac{3}{20}$.

To convert a percent to a decimal, follow these steps:

1) Write the percent over 100 because percent means "per one hundred." So, 15% can be written as $\frac{15}{100}$.

2) 15 divided by 100 equals 0.15, so 15% = 0.15. In other words, when converting from a percent to a decimal, drop the percent sign and move the decimal two places to the left.

Example 2

Write 24.36% as a fraction and then as a decimal. Explain how you made these conversions.

24.36% written as a fraction is $\frac{24.36}{100}$, or $\frac{2436}{10,000}$, which reduces to $\frac{609}{2500}$. 24.36% written as a decimal is 0.2436. Recall that

dividing by 100 moves the decimal two places to the left.

Example 3

Convert $\frac{4}{5}$ to a decimal and to a percent.

To convert a fraction to a decimal, simply divide the numerator by the denominator in the fraction. The numerator is the top number in the fraction and the denominator is the bottom number in a fraction. So $\frac{4}{5} = 4 \div 5 = 0.80 = 0.8$.

Percent means "per hundred." $\frac{4 \cdot 20}{5 \cdot 20} = \frac{80}{100}$ = 80%.

Example 4

Convert $3\frac{2}{5}$ to a decimal and to a percent.

The mixed number $3\frac{2}{5}$ has a whole number and a fractional part. The fractional part, namely $\frac{2}{5}$, can be written as a decimal by dividing 5 into 2, which gives 0.4. Adding the whole to the part gives 3.4. Alternatively, note that

$$3\frac{2}{5} = 3\frac{4}{10} = 3.4$$

To change a decimal to a percent, multiply it by 100.

3.4(100) = 340%. Notice that this percentage is greater than 100%. This makes sense because the original mixed number $3\frac{2}{5}$ is greater than 1.

Product with decimals

When numbers are multiplied, the resulting number is the product. For example, the product of 2 and 4 is 8 because 2 × 4 = 8. When finding the product of numbers containing decimals, it is often helpful to multiply the numbers as if neither contains a decimal and then to adjust the product afterwards.

For instance,

$$\begin{array}{r} 25 \\ \times\ \ 4 \\ \hline 100 \end{array}$$

In order to change 2.5 to a whole number to make multiplying easier, you essentially multiply it by ten, which moves the decimal one place to the right. Because 25 is ten times 2.5, the product of 25 and 4 (100) is ten times the product of 2.5 and 4. To adjust for the initial change, you must divide the product by ten, which moves the decimal one place back to the left. So, the product of 2.5 and 4 is 10 (or 10.0).

Percentage

Example 1
What is 30% of 120?

The word "of" indicates multiplication, so 30% of 120 is found by multiplying 30% by 120. First, change 30% to a fraction or decimal. Recall that "percent" means per hundred, so 30% = $\frac{30}{100}$ = 0.30. 120 times 0.3 is 36.

Example 2
What is 150% of 20?

150% of 20 is found by multiplying 150% by 20. First, change 150% to a fraction or decimal. Recall that "percent" means per hundred, so 150% = $\frac{150}{100}$ = 1.50. So, (1.50)(20) = 30. Notice that 30 is greater than the original number of 20. This makes sense because you are finding a number that is more than 100% of the original number.

Example 3
According to a hospital survey, 82% of nurses were highly satisfied at their job. Of 145 nurses, how many were highly satisfied?

82% of 145 = 0.82 · 145 = 118.9. Because you can't have 0.9 of a person, the answer is "about 119 nurses are highly satisfied with their jobs."

Example 4
What is 14.5% of 96?

Change 14.5% to a decimal before multiplying. 0.145 · 96 = 13.92. Notice that 13.92 is much smaller than the original number of 96. This makes sense because you are finding a small percentage of the original number.

Example 5
Find 275% of 33.

Change 275% to a decimal before multiplying: 275% of 33 = (275%)(33) = (2.75)(33) = 90.75. Notice that 90.75 is greater than the original number of 33. This makes sense because you are finding a number that is more than 100% of the original number.

Mathematical reasoning and computational procedures

Example 1
By what percentage does $\frac{3}{4}$ exceed $\frac{1}{3}$?

$$\frac{\text{new fraction} - \text{original fraction}}{\text{original fraction}} \cdot 100\% =$$
percent increase.
$$\frac{\frac{3}{4} - \frac{1}{3}}{\frac{1}{3}} \cdot 100\% = \frac{\frac{5}{12}}{\frac{1}{3}} \cdot 100\% = \frac{5}{12} \cdot \frac{3}{1} \cdot 100\% = \frac{15}{12} \cdot 100\% = 125\%.$$

Example 2
A patient's age is thirteen more than half of 60. How old is the patient?

"More than" indicates addition, and "of" indicates multiplication. The expression can be written as "1/2(60) + 13". So, the patient's age is equal to $\frac{1}{2}$(60) + 13 = 30 + 13 = 43. The patient is 43 years old.

Simplifying

<u>Example 1</u>
How to simplify:

$$\frac{\frac{2}{5}}{\frac{4}{7}}$$

Dividing a fraction by a fraction may appear tricky, but it's not if you write out your steps carefully. Follow these steps to divide a fraction by a fraction.
Step 1: Rewrite the problem as a multiplication problem. Dividing by a fraction is the same as multiplying by its reciprocal, also known as its multiplicative inverse. The product of a number and its reciprocal is 1. Because $\frac{4}{7}$ times $\frac{7}{4}$ is 1, these numbers are reciprocals. Note that reciprocals can be found by simply interchanging the numerators and denominators. So, rewriting the problem as a multiplication problem gives
$\frac{2}{5} \times \frac{7}{4}$.
Step 2: Perform multiplication of the fractions by multiplying the numerators by each other and the denominators by each other. In other words, multiply across the top and then multiply across the bottom.

$$\frac{2}{5} \times \frac{7}{4} = \frac{2 \times 7}{5 \times 4} = \frac{14}{20}$$

Step 3: Make sure the fraction is reduced to lowest terms. Both 14 and 20 can be divided by 2.
$\frac{14}{20} = \frac{14 \div 2}{20 \div 2} = \frac{7}{10}$
The answer is $\frac{7}{10}$.

<u>Example 2</u>
How to simplify:

$$\frac{1}{4} + \frac{3}{6}$$

Fractions with common denominators can be easily added or subtracted. Recall that the denominator is the bottom number in the fraction and that the numerator is the top number in the fraction.
The denominators of $\frac{1}{4}$ and $\frac{3}{6}$ are 4 and 6, respectively. The lowest common denominator of 4 and 6 is 12 because 12 is the least common multiple of 4 (multiples 4, 8, 12, 16, …) and 6 (multiples 6, 12, 18, 24, …). Convert each fraction to its equivalent with the newly found common denominator of 12.
$\frac{1 \times 3}{4 \times 3} = \frac{3}{12}; \frac{3 \times 2}{6 \times 2} = \frac{6}{12}$.
Now that the fractions have the same denominator, you can add them.
$\frac{3}{12} + \frac{6}{12} = \frac{9}{12}$.
Be sure to write your answer in lowest terms. Both 9 and 12 can be divided by 3, so the answer is $\frac{3}{4}$.

<u>Example 3</u>
How to simplify:

$$\frac{7}{8} - \frac{8}{16}$$

Fractions with common denominators can be easily added or subtracted. Recall that the denominator is the bottom number in the fraction and that the numerator is the top number in the fraction.
The denominators of $\frac{7}{8}$ and $\frac{8}{16}$ are 8 and 16, respectively. The lowest common denominator of 8 and 16 is 16 because 16 is the least common multiple of 8 (multiples 8, 16, 24 …) and 16 (multiples 16, 32, 48, …). Convert each fraction to its equivalent with the newly found common denominator of 16.
$\frac{7 \times 2}{8 \times 2} = \frac{14}{16}; \frac{8 \times 1}{16 \times 1} = \frac{8}{16}$.
Now that the fractions have the same denominator, you can subtract them.
$\frac{14}{16} - \frac{8}{16} = \frac{6}{16}$.

Be sure to write your answer in lowest terms. Both 6 and 16 can be divided by 2, so the answer is $\frac{3}{8}$.

Example 4
How to simplify:
$$\frac{1}{2} + (3(\frac{3}{4}) - 2) + 4^2$$

When simplifying expressions, first perform operations within groups. Within the set of parentheses are multiplication and subtraction operations. Perform the multiplication first to get $\frac{1}{2} + (\frac{9}{4} - 2) + 4^2$.
Then, subtract two to obtain $\frac{1}{2} + \frac{1}{4} + 4^2$.
Next, evaluate the exponent: $\frac{1}{2} + \frac{1}{4} + 16$.
Finally, perform addition from left to right.
$$\frac{1}{2} + \frac{1}{4} + 16 \rightarrow \frac{2}{4} + \frac{1}{4} + \frac{64}{4} = \frac{67}{4}.$$

Example 5
How to simplify:
$$0.22 + 0.5^2 - (5.5 + 3.3 \div 3)$$

First, evaluate the terms in the parentheses $(5.5 + 3.3 \div 3)$ using order of operations. $3.3 \div 3 = 1.1$, and $5.5 + 1.1 = 6.6$. Rewrite the problem: $0.22 + 0.5^2 - 6.6$. Next, evaluate the exponent of $0.5^2 = 0.5 \times 0.5 = 0.25$.
Rewrite the problem: $0.22 + 0.25 - 6.6$.
Finally, add and subtract from left to right.
$0.22 + 0.25 = 0.47 \rightarrow 0.47 - 6.6 = -6.13$.
The answer is -6.13.

Example 6
How to simplify:
$$\frac{3}{2} + (4(0.5) - 0.75) + 2^2$$

First, simplify within the parentheses:
$\frac{3}{2} + (4(0.5) - 0.75) + 2^2$
$\frac{3}{2} + (2 - 0.75) + 2^2$
$\frac{3}{2} + 1.25 + 2^2$

Next, evaluate the exponent.
$\frac{3}{2} + 1.25 + 4$
Finally, perform addition from left to right. Change the fraction to a decimal or convert all the numbers to fractions with common denominators.
$1.5 + 1.25 + 4 = 6.75$ or $6\frac{3}{4}$
Finally, perform addition from left to right. Change the fraction to a decimal or convert all the numbers to fractions with common denominators.
$1.5 + 1.25 + 4 = 6.75$ or $6\frac{3}{4}$

Example 7
How to simplify:
$$1.45 + 1.5^2 + (6 - 9 \div 2) + 45$$

First, evaluate the terms in the parentheses using proper order of operations.
$1.45 + 1.5^2 + (6 - 9 \div 2) + 45$
$1.45 + 1.5^2 + (6 - 4.5) + 45$
$1.45 + 1.5^2 + 1.5 + 45$
Next, evaluate the exponent.
$1.45 + 2.25 + 1.5 + 45$
Finally, add from left to right.
$1.45 + 2.25 + 1.5 + 45 = 50.2$

Word problems

Example 1
A patient was given pain medicine at a dosage of 0.22 grams. The patient's dosage was then increased to 0.80 grams. By how much was the patient's dosage increased?

The first step is to determine what operation (addition, subtraction, multiplication, or division) the problem requires. Notice the key words and phrases "by how much" and "increased." "Increased" means that you go from a smaller amount to a larger amount. This change can be found by subtracting the smaller amount from the larger amount: 0.80 grams – 0.22 grams = 0.58 grams.

Remember to line up the decimal when subtracting.

```
  0.80
- 0.22
  0.58
```

Example 2

At a hospital, $\frac{3}{4}$ of the 100 beds are occupied today. Yesterday, $\frac{4}{5}$ of the 100 beds were occupied. On which day and by how much more were more of the hospital beds occupied?

First, find the actual number of beds that were occupied each day. To do so, multiply the fraction of beds occupied by the number of beds available:
Actual number of beds occupied = fraction of beds occupied × number of beds available
Today: Actual number of beds occupied = $\frac{3}{4}$ × 100.

$$\frac{3}{4} \times \frac{100}{1} = \frac{3 \times 100}{4 \times 1} = \frac{300}{4}$$

Then, write the fraction in lowest terms.

$$\frac{300}{4} \div \frac{4}{4} = \frac{75}{1} = 75.$$

Today, 75 beds are occupied.
Yesterday: Actual number of beds occupied = $\frac{4}{5}$ × 100.

$$\frac{4}{5} \times \frac{100}{1} = \frac{4 \times 100}{5 \times 1} = \frac{400}{5}$$

Then, write the fraction in lowest terms.

$$\frac{400}{5} \div \frac{5}{5} = \frac{80}{1} = 80.$$

Yesterday, 80 beds were occupied.
The difference in the number of beds occupied is 80 – 75 = 5 beds.
Therefore, five more beds were occupied yesterday than today.

Example 3

A patient complaining of fatigue and weight gain was diagnosed with hypothyroidism and was prescribed 125 mcg of medication. Three months later, her symptoms had improved, and her thyroid stimulation hormone (TSH) level was found to be 0.5 mIU/L. The doctor reduced the patient's thyroid medication dosage to 100 mcg, after which the patient's TSH level was found to be 1.5 mIU/L, which is within the normal range. By what percentage did the doctor reduce the patient's thyroid medication?

In this problem you must determine which information is necessary to answer the question. The question asks by what percentage the doctor reduced the patient's thyroid medication dosage. Find the two dosage amounts and perform subtraction to find their difference. The first dosage amount is 125 mcg. The second dosage amount is 100 mcg. Therefore, the difference is 125 mcg – 100 mcg = 25 mcg. The percentage reduction can then be calculated as $\frac{change}{original} = \frac{25\ mcg}{125\ mcg} = \frac{1}{5} = 20\%$.

Example 4

In a hospital emergency room, there are 4 nurses for every 12 patients. What is the ratio of nurses to patients? If the nurse-to-patient ratio remains constant, how many nurses must be present to care for 24 patients?

The ratio of nurses to patients can be written as 4 to 12, 4:12, or $\frac{4}{12}$. Because four and twelve have a common factor of four, the ratio should be reduced to 1:3, which means that there is one nurse present for every three patients. If this ratio remains constant, there must be eight nurses present to care for 24 patients.

Example 5

In an intensive care unit, the nurse-to-patient ratio is 1:2. If seven nurses are on duty, how many patients are currently in the ICU?

Use proportional reasoning or set up a proportion to solve. Because there are twice as many patients as nurses, there must be fourteen patients when seven nurses are on duty. Setting up and solving a proportion gives the same result:

$$\frac{\text{number of nurses}}{\text{number of patients}} = \frac{1}{2}$$

$$= \frac{7}{\text{number of patients}}$$

Represent the unknown number of patients as the variable x.

$$\frac{1}{2} = \frac{7}{x}$$

To solve for x, cross multiply:
$1 \cdot x = 7 \cdot 2$, so $x = 14$.

Example 6
During a shift, a new nurse spent five hours of her time observing procedures, three hours working in the oncology department, and four hours doing paperwork. During the next shift, she spent four hours observing procedures, six hours in the oncology department, and two hours doing paperwork. What was the percent change for each task between the two shifts?

The three tasks are observing procedures, working in the oncology department, and doing paperwork. To find the amount of change, compare the first amount with the second amount for each task. Then, write this difference as a percentage compared to the initial amount.
Amount of change for observing procedures: 5 hours – 4 hours = 1 hour.
The percent of change is $\frac{\text{amount of change}}{\text{original amount}} \cdot$ 100%. $\frac{1 \text{ hour}}{5 \text{ hours}} \cdot 100\% = 20\%$. The nurse spent 20% less time observing procedures on her second shift than on her first.
Amount of change for working in the oncology department: 6 hours – 3 hours = 3 hours.
The percent of change is $\frac{\text{amount of change}}{\text{original amount}} \cdot$ 100%. $\frac{3 \text{ hours}}{3 \text{ hours}} \cdot 100\% = 100\%$. The nurse spent 100% more time (or twice as much time) working in the oncology

department during her second shift than she did in her first.
Amount of change for doing paperwork: 4 hours – 2 hours = 2 hours.
The percent of change is $\frac{\text{amount of change}}{\text{original amount}} \cdot$ 100%. $\frac{2 \text{ hours}}{4 \text{ hours}} \cdot 100\% = 50\%$. The nurse spent 50% less time (or half as much time) working on paperwork during her second shift than she did in her first.

Example 7
A patient's heart beat 422 times over the course of six minutes. About how many times did the patient's heart beat during each minute?

"About how many" indicates that you need to estimate the solution. In this case, look at the numbers you are given. 422 can be rounded down to 420, which is easily divisible by 6. A good estimate is $420 \div 6 = 70$ beats per minute. More accurately, the patient's heart rate was just over 70 beats per minute since his heart actually beat a little more than 420 times in six minutes

Example 8
At a hospital, 40% of the nurses work in labor and delivery. If 20 nurses work in labor and delivery, how many nurses work at the hospital?

To answer this problem, first think about the number of nurses that work at the hospital. Will it be more or less than the number of nurses who work in a specific department such as labor and delivery? More nurses work at the hospital, so the number you find to answer this question will be greater than 20.
40% of the nurses are labor and delivery nurses. "Of" indicates multiplication, and words like "is" and "are" indicate equivalence. Translating the problem into a mathematical sentence gives
$40\% \cdot n = 20$, where n represents the total number of nurses. Solving for n gives

- 24 -

$n = \dfrac{20}{40\%} = \dfrac{20}{0.40} = 50.$

Fifty nurses work at the hospital.

Example 9

A patient was given 40 mg of a certain medicine. Later, the patient's dosage was increased to 45 mg. What was the percent increase in his medication? To find the percent increase, first compare the original and increased amounts. The original amount was 40 mg, and the increased amount is 45 mg, so the dosage of medication was increased by 5 mg (45 − 40 = 5). Note, however, that the question asks not by how much the dosage increased but by what *percentage* it increased. Percent increase

$= \dfrac{new\ amount\ -original\ amount}{original\ amount} \cdot 100\%.$

So, $\dfrac{45\ mg - 40\ mg}{40\ mg} \cdot 100\% = \dfrac{5}{40} \cdot 100\% = 0.125 \cdot 100\% \approx 12.5\%$

The percent increase is approximately 12.5%.

Example 10

A patient was given 100 mg of a medicine every two hours. How much medication will the patient receive in four hours?

Using proportional reasoning, since four hours is twice as long as two hours, the patient will receive twice as much medication, 2·100 mg = 200 mg, within that time period.

To write an equation, first, write the amount of medicine per 2 hours as a ratio.

$$\dfrac{100\ mg}{2\ hours}$$

Next create a proportion to relate the different time increments of 2 hours and 4 hours.

$\dfrac{100\ mg}{2\ hours} = \dfrac{x\ mg}{4\ hours}$, where x is the amount of medicine the patient receives in four hours. Make sure to keep the same units in either the numerator or denominator. In this case the numerator units must be mg for both ratios and the denominator units must be hours for both ratios.

Use cross multiplication and division to solve for x.

$\dfrac{100\ mg}{2\ hours} = \dfrac{x\ mg}{4\ hours}$

$100(4) = 2(x)$

$400 = 2x$

$400 \div 2 = 2x \div 2$

$200 = x$

Therefore, the patient receives 200 mg every four hours.

Example 11

Jane ate lunch at a local restaurant. She ordered a $4.99 appetizer, $12.50 entrée, and $1.25 soda. If she wants to tip her server 20%, how much money will she spend in all?

To find total amount, first find the sum of the items she ordered from the menu and then add 20% of this sum to the total.
In other words:
$4.99 + $12.50 + $1.25 = $18.74.
Then 20% of $18.74 is (20%)($18.74) = (0.20)($18.74) = $3.75.
So, the total she spends is cost of the meal plus the tip or $18.74 + $3.75 = $22.49.
Another way to find this sum is to multiply 120% by the cost of the meal.
$18.74(120%) = $18.74(1.20) = $22.49.

Example 12

A patient was given 100 mg of a certain medicine. The patient's dosage was later decreased to 88mg. What was the percent decrease?

The medication was decreased by 12 mg (100 mg - 88 mg = 12 mg). To find by what percent the medication was decreased, this change must be written as a percentage when compared to the original amount.

In other words, $\dfrac{original\ amount\ -new\ amount}{original\ amount} \cdot$ 100% = percent decrease

So $\dfrac{12\ mg}{100\ mg} \cdot 100\% = 0.12 \cdot 100\% = 12\%.$

The percent decrease is 12%.

Example 13
A patient was given blood pressure medicine at a dosage of 2 grams. The patient's dosage was then decreased to 0.45 grams. By how much was the patient's dosage decreased?

The decrease is represented by the difference between the two amounts: 2 grams – 0.45 grams = 1.55 grams. Remember to line up the decimal point before subtracting.

```
  2.00
- 0.45
  1.55
```

Example 14
Two weeks ago, $\frac{2}{3}$ of the 60 patients at a hospital were male. Last week, $\frac{3}{6}$ of the 80 patients were male. During which week were there more male patients?

First, you need to find the number of male patients that were in the hospital each week. You are given this amount in terms of fractions. To find the actual number of male patients, multiply the fraction of male patients by the number of patients in the hospital.
Actual number of male patients = fraction of male patients × total number of patients.
Two weeks ago: Actual number of male patients $= \frac{2}{3} \times 60$.
$\frac{2}{3} \times \frac{60}{1} = \frac{2 \times 60}{3 \times 1} = \frac{120}{3} = 40$.
Two weeks ago, 40 of the patients were male.
Last week: Actual number of male patients $= \frac{3}{6} \times 80$.
$\frac{3}{6} \times \frac{80}{1} = \frac{3 \times 80}{6 \times 1} = \frac{240}{6} = 40$.
Last week, 40 of the patients were male. The number of male patients was the same both weeks.

Example 15
At a hospital, for every 20 female patients there are 15 male patients. This same patient ratio happens to exist at another hospital. If there are 100 female patients at the second hospital, how many male patients are there?

One way to find the number of male patients is to set up and solve a proportion.
$$\frac{number\ of\ female\ patients}{number\ of\ male\ patients} = \frac{20}{15} = \frac{100}{number\ of\ male\ patients}.$$
Represent the unknown number of male patients as the variable x.
$\frac{20}{15} = \frac{100}{x}$.
Follow these steps to solve for x.
1) Cross multiply. $20 \times x = 15 \times 100$.
$20x = 1500$
2) Divide each side of the equation by 20.
$x = 75$
Or, notice that
$\frac{20 \cdot 5}{15 \cdot 5} = \frac{100}{75}$, so $x = 75$.

Example 16
In a performance review, an employee received a score of 70 out of 100 for efficiency and 90 out of 100 for meeting project deadlines. Six months later, the employee received a score of 65 out of 100 for efficiency and 96 out of 100 for meeting project deadlines. What was the percent change for each score on the performance review?

To find the percent change, compare the first amount with the second amount for each score; then, write this difference as a percentage compared to the initial amount. Or, write the original amounts as percentages and then subtract.
Percent change for efficiency score:
70% – 65% = 5%.
The employee's efficiency decreased by 5%.
Percent change for meeting project deadlines score:

96% − 90% = 6%
The employee increased his ability to meet project deadlines by 6%.

Example 17

A patient's total bill is about $128 for the same procedure repeated each month for 5 months. About how much does the procedure cost?

"About how much" indicates that you need to estimate the solution. In this case, look at the numbers you are given which are $128 and 5. 128 can be rounded up to 130 which is easily divisible by 5. So a good estimate is 130 ÷ 5 = $26 per procedure. More accurately, the procedure costs a little less than $26.

Subtracting fractions

Fractions with common denominators can be easily added or subtracted. Recall that the denominator is the bottom number in the fraction and that the numerator is the top number in the fraction. For example, subtract $\frac{1}{5}$ from $\frac{3}{4}$:

The denominators of $\frac{3}{4}$ and $\frac{1}{5}$ are 4 and 5, respectively. The lowest common denominator of 4 and 5 is 20 because 20 is the least common multiple of 4 (multiples 4, 8, 16, 20 …) and 5 (multiples 5, 10, 15, 20, …). Convert each fraction to its equivalent with the newly found common denominator of 20.
$\frac{3\times5}{4\times5} = \frac{15}{20}, \frac{1\times4}{5\times4} = \frac{4}{20}.$
Now that the fractions have the same denominator, you can subtract them.
$\frac{15}{20} - \frac{4}{20} = \frac{11}{20}.$

Subtracting with regrouping

Example 1

Demonstrate how to subtract 189 from 525 using regrouping.

First, set up the subtraction problem:
```
  525
- 189
```
Notice that the numbers in the ones and tens columns of 525 are smaller than the numbers in the ones and tens columns of 189. This means you will need to use regrouping to perform subtraction.
```
  5  2  5
- 1  8  9
```
To subtract 9 from 5 in the ones column you will need to borrow from the 2 in the tens columns:
```
  5  1  15
- 1  8   9
         6
```
Next, to subtract 8 from 1 in the tens column you will need to borrow from the 5 in the hundreds column:
```
  4  11  15
- 1   8   9
      3   6
```
Last, subtract the 1 from the 4 in the hundreds column:
```
  4  11  15
- 1   8   9
  3   3   6
```

Example 2

Demonstrate how to subtract 477 from 620 using regrouping.

First, set up the subtraction problem:
```
  620
- 477
```
Notice that the numbers in the ones and tens columns of 620 are smaller than the numbers in the ones and tens columns of 477. This means you will need to use regrouping to perform subtraction.
```
  6  2  0
- 4  7  7
```
To subtract 7 from 0 in the ones column you will need to borrow from the 2 in the tens column.
```
  6  1  10
- 4  7   7
         3
```

Next, to subtract 7 from the 1 that's still in the tens column you will need to borrow from the 6 in the hundreds column.

```
  5  11 10
- 4  7  7
     4  3
```

Lastly, subtract 4 from the 5 remaining in the hundreds column to get:

```
  5  11 10
- 4  7  7
  1  4  3
```

Calculation of salary after deductions

Example 1

Before taxes, a monthly paycheck was $2,160. However, the following deductions were taken from the paycheck: Federal Withholding, $154; Social Security, $90.72; Medicare $31.22; and State Withholding, $126.20. What is actual amount of the paycheck after these deductions?

Notice the key words in the problem: the words "deduction" and "from" indicate subtraction. To determine the amount of the paycheck after the deductions, or expenses, use either of these methods.
Method 1: Add all the deductions. Then, subtract this amount from the original amount.
Total Deductions = $154 + $90.72 + $31.22 + $126.20 = $402.14
Subtract this total amount from the original amount. $2,160 - $402.14 = $1,757.86.
Method 2: Subtract each amount from the original amount.
$2,160 - $154 - $90.72 - $31.22 - $126.20 = $1,757.86

Example 2

Before taxes, a monthly paycheck was $787.57. However, the following deductions were taken from the paycheck: Federal Withholding, $78.42; Social Security, $36.99; Medicare, $7.04; and State Withholding, $45.86. What is amount of the paycheck after these deductions?

Deductions, or expenses, are subtracted from the original amount. There are two ways to answer this problem.
Method 1: Add all the deductions. Then subtract this amount from the original amount.
Total Deductions = $78.42 + $36.99 + $7.04 + $45.86 = $168.31
Subtract this total amount from the original amount. $787.57 - $168.31 = $619.26.
Method 2: Subtract each amount from the original amount.
$787.57 - $78.42 - $36.99 - $7.04 - $45.86 = $619.26

Calculation of balance after transactions

Example 1
Two weeks ago, a checking account had a balance of $7,809.45. The transactions for the last two weeks are shown in table below.

Water Bill	$36.78	Expense
Pay Check	$2,891.45	Income
Cell Phone Bill	$98.99	Expense
Credit Card Bill	$375.17	Expense
Refund for returned clothing items	$45.28	Refund

What is the new account balance after these transactions?

When reconciling a checking account balance, you need to know what operation (addition or subtraction) to use for each transaction. An expense is a deduction from the account balance. Therefore, you subtract the expense amount from the account balance. A transaction labeled "income" means that you are adding the amount to your account balance. Lastly, a refund means that you are receiving, or adding money back, to your account

To find the new account balance, perform the following operations:

$7,809.45 - $36.78 + $2,891.45 - $98.99 - $375.17 + $45.28 = $10,235.24

Example 2

Two months ago, a checking account had a balance of $4,009.67. The transactions for the last two months are shown in table below.

Electric Bill	$189.45	Expense
Paycheck	$1,000.31	Income
Internet Bill	$68.77	Expense
Paycheck	$1,000.31	Income
Sold items on Ebay	$201.55	Income

What is the new account balance after these transactions?

When reconciling a checking account balance, you need to know what operation (addition or subtraction) to use for each transaction. An expense is a deduction from the account balance. Therefore, you would subtract the expense amount from the account balance. An income is added to the account balance.

To find the new account balance, perform the following operations:

$4,009.67 - $189.45 + $1,000.31 - $68.77 + $1,000.31 + $201.55 = $5953.62

Solving for x in a proportion

Solve for x in this proportion: $\frac{10}{15} = \frac{x}{30}$.

There are two ways to solve for x.

Method 1: Cross multiply; then, solve for x.

$$\frac{10}{15} = \frac{x}{30}$$

$10(30) = 15(x)$

$300 = 15x$

$300 \div 15 = 15x \div 15$

$x = 20$

Method 2: Notice that 30 is twice as much as 15, so x should be twice as much as 10. Therefore, $x = 10 \times 2 = 20$.

Absolute value

The absolute value of a number is its distance from zero on a number line. Because a distance is represented by a positive number, the absolute value of a number will always be positive. The absolute value is indicated by two vertical lines on either side of the number: $|\#|$. For example, $|-10| = 10$; $|4.48| = 4.48$; $|-78\%| = 78\%$; $\left|\frac{2}{3}\right| = \frac{2}{3}$; $\left|\frac{-7}{12}\right| = \frac{7}{12}$; $|-30.54\%| = 30.54\%$.

Roman numerals

The Roman numeral I represents 1, V represents 5, X represents 10, C represents 100, and M represents 1,000. IX means "one number before ten." The number before ten is nine, so IX = 9. The Roman numeral XI indicates "one number after ten," or 11. XV means "five numbers after ten," or 15. CM means "100 numbers before 1000," or 900.

Decimal placement in a product

What is 3.52 × 5? How did you find this answer?

When finding the product of numbers containing decimals, it is often helpful to multiply the numbers as if neither contains a decimal and then to adjust the product afterwards. For instance, 352 × 5 = 1760.

In order to change 3.52 to a whole number to make multiplying easier, you essentially multiply it by 100, which moves the decimal two places to the right. Because 352 is 100 times 3.52, the product of 352 and 5 (1760) is 100 times the product of 3.52 and 5. To adjust for the initial change, you must divide the product by 100, which moves the decimal two places back to the left. So, the product of 3.52 and 5 is 17.6 (or 17.60). An easier way to think about this may be to count the total number of digits after each decimal in the original problem and make sure the answer contains the same number of digits after its decimal. Since there are two numbers after a decimal in the problem, there should be two numbers after the decimal in the answer. So, the answer must be 17.60. (Note that a decimal was inserted in the number 1760 such that there are two numbers, namely the six and zero, after the decimal in the adjusted answer just as there are two numbers, namely the five and two, after a decimal in the problem.) It is also worthwhile to ensure that your answer makes sense. 3.52 is between 3 and 4, so 3.52 × 5 should be between 3 × 5 and 4 × 5. Indeed, 17.6 is between 15 and 20, so it is a sensible answer.

Equivalent ratios

Example
Write two ratios that are equivalent to 5:25.

5:25 can be reduced to 1:5. Any ratio in which the second term is five times the first is equivalent to the given ratio. Two additional examples are 3:15 and 25:125.

Rational numbers from least to greatest

Order the following rational numbers from least to greatest: 0.55, 17%, $\sqrt{25}$, $\frac{64}{4}$, $\frac{25}{50}$, 3.

The term "rational" simply means that the number can be expressed as a ratio, or fraction. The set of rational numbers includes integers, of which whole numbers are a subset, because these numbers can be written as ratios. Notice that each of the numbers in the problem can be written as fractions:

$\sqrt{25} = 5 = \frac{5}{1}$

$0.55 = \frac{55}{100}$

$17\% = 0.17 = \frac{17}{100}$

To order the numbers from least to greatest, compare their values.

Notice that $\frac{64}{4}$ is equal to 16, and $\frac{25}{50}$ can be written as $\frac{1}{2}$.

So, the answer is 17%, $\frac{25}{50}$, 0.55, 3, $\sqrt{25}$, $\frac{64}{4}$.

Rational numbers from greatest to least

Order the following rational numbers from greatest to least: 0.3, 27%, $\sqrt{100}$, $\frac{72}{9}$, $\frac{1}{9}$, 4.5

The term "rational" simply means that the number can be expressed as a ratio, or fraction. The set of rational numbers includes integers, of which whole numbers are a subset, because these numbers can be written as ratios. Notice that each of the numbers in the problem can be written as fractions:

$\sqrt{100} = 10 = \frac{10}{1}$

$0.3 = \frac{3}{10}$

$27\% = 0.27 = \frac{27}{100}$

Also notice that $\frac{72}{9}$ is equal to 8 and that $\frac{1}{9}$ is approximately 0.11.

So, the answer is $\sqrt{100}$, $\frac{72}{9}$, 4.5, 0.3, 27%, $\frac{1}{9}$.

Algebraic Applications

Equations with one unknown

<u>Example 1</u>

$\frac{45\%}{12\%} = \frac{15\%}{x}$. Solve for x.

First, cross multiply; then, solve for x:

$\frac{45\%}{12\%} = \frac{15\%}{x}$

$\frac{0.45}{0.12} = \frac{0.15}{x}$.

$0.45(x) = 0.12(0.15)$

$0.45\,x = 0.0180$

$0.45x \div 0.45 = 0.0180 \div 0.45$

$x = 0.04 = 4\%$

Alternatively, notice that $\frac{45\% \div 3}{12\% \div 3} = \frac{15\%}{4\%}$. So, $x = 4\%$.

<u>Example 2</u>

How do you solve for x in the proportion $\frac{0.50}{2} = \frac{1.50}{x}$?

First, cross multiply; then, solve for x.

$\frac{0.50}{2} = \frac{1.50}{x}$.

$0.50(x) = 2(1.50)$

$0.50x = 3$

$0.50x \div 0.50 = 3 \div 0.50$

$x = 6$

Or, notice that $\frac{0.50 \cdot 3}{2 \cdot 3} = \frac{1.50}{6}$, so $x = 6$.

<u>Example 3</u>

$\frac{40}{8} = \frac{x}{24}$. Find x.

One way to solve for x is to first cross multiply.

$\frac{40}{8} = \frac{x}{24}$.

$40(24) = 8(x)$

$960 = 8x$

$960 \div 8 = 8x \div 8$

$x = 120$

Or, notice that:

$\frac{40 \cdot 3}{8 \cdot 3} = \frac{120}{24}$, so $x = 120$

<u>Example 4</u>

$x = \frac{1}{4} + 70\%$. Write your answer as a percent and as a fraction in lowest terms.

The key is to write the two values in the same format. You can write both of them as percents and then perform addition, or you can write both of them as fractions and then perform addition.
Method 1: Write both numbers as percents and then perform addition.
To convert $\frac{1}{4}$ to a percent simply divide the numerator by the denominator in the fraction and then multiply by 100%. $\frac{1}{4} =$ 0.25. Then 0.25(100%) = 25%.
Then perform addition: x = 25% + 70% = 95%.

$95\% = \frac{95}{100} = \frac{19}{20}$.

Method 2: Write both numbers as fractions and then perform addition.

$70\% = \frac{70}{100} = \frac{7}{10}$.

$x = \frac{7}{10} + \frac{1}{4} = \frac{14}{20} + \frac{5}{20} = \frac{19}{20}$.

$\frac{19}{20} = \frac{95}{100} = 95\%$.

Polynomials and monomials

<u>Example 1</u>

Simplify $10c^2 + 25c - 3c^2 - 10$.

This is an example of a polynomial. To perform addition and subtraction on a polynomial you must first identify "like" terms. "Like" terms have the same variable with the same exponent. For example $10c^2$ and $- 3c^2$ are "like" terms because they both have the variable c with exponent of 2, so they both have c^2. After you identify "like" terms, add or subtract their coefficients.

$10c^2 - 3c^2 = (10 - 3)\,c^2 = 7c^2$

There are no other "like" terms in the polynomial, so the answer written in descending powers of c is $7c^2 + 25c - 10$.

Example 2
Simplify $4b(2b^3 - 5f^4 + 3b^2 + 7)$.

This is an example of multiplying monomial and polynomial terms. Use the distributive property by multiplying the term $4b$ by each term in the parentheses:
$4b(2b^3) - 4b(5f^4) + 4b(3b^2) + 4b(7)$
When multiplying monomials, first multiply the coefficients: $(4 \times 2)(b \times b^3) - (4 \times 5)(b \times f^4) + (4 \times 3)(b \times b^2) + (4 \times 7)(b)$
When multiplying powers with the same base, add their exponents:
$8b^{(1+3)} - 20bf^4 + 12b^{(1+2)} + 28b$
$8b^4 - 20bf^4 + 12b^3 + 28b$
Notice that the exponents for b and f can't be combined since the variables are not the same.

Example 3
What is $6x^8y^3z$ divided by $3x^3y^5z^2$?

This is an example of dividing the monomials $6x^8y^3z$ and $3x^3y^5z^2$: When simplifying
$6x^8y^3z \div 3x^3y^5z^2$, first divide the coefficients of the variables: $6 \div 3 = 2$.
For each variable, subtract the exponent in the second term from the exponent in the first term.
$x^{8-3} = x^5$
$y^{3-5} = y^{-2}$
$z^{1-2} = z^{-1}$ Note: $z = z^1$.
The resulting $2x^5 y^{-2} z^{-1}$ should be written with only positive exponents. Because $y^{-2} = \frac{1}{y^2}$ and $z^{-1} = \frac{1}{z}$, $2x^5 y^{-2} z^{-1}$ is the same as $\frac{2x^5}{y^2z}$.

Translating

Words to mathematical expression
Write "four less than twice x" as a mathematical expression.

Remember that an expression does not have an equals sign. "Less" indicates subtraction, and "twice" indicates multiplication by two. Four less than $2x$ is $2x - 4$. Notice how this is different than $4 - 2x$. You can plug in values for x to see how these expressions would yield different values.

Words to mathematical sentence
Translate "three hundred twenty-five increased by six times $3x$ equals three hundred forty-three" into a mathematical sentence.

The key words and phrases are "increased by," "times," and "equals." Three hundred twenty-five increased by six times $3x$ equals three hundred forty-three:
$$325 + 6(3x) = 343.$$

The mathematical sentence is $325 + 6(3x) = 343$.

Words to inequality
Write an inequality that represents "64 plus $25f$ is less than or equal to 23 plus the quantity x minus 44."

The key words and phrases are "plus," "less than or equal to," "the quantity," and "minus." The first part of the number sentence is *64 plus 25f*. "Plus" indicates addition. So this can be written as $64 + 25f$ which will go on the left hand side of the inequality sign.
"Less than or equal to" is represented with the inequality symbol $\leq$.
The second part of the number sentence is *23 plus the quantity x minus 44*. "Plus" indicates addition. "The quantity x minus 44" means that 44 must be subtracted from x before it is added to the 23; in other words, the "x minus 44" needs to be grouped together inside parentheses. All together, this can be written as $23 + (x - 44)$, which goes on the right hand side of the inequality sign.
The final answer is $64 + 25f \leq 23 + (x - 44)$.

<u>Mathematical expression to a phrase</u>
Write a phrase which represents this mathematical expression: $75 - 3t + 14^2$.

Because there are many words which indicate various operations, there are several ways to write this expression, including "seventy-five minus three times *t* plus fourteen squared."

Data Interpretation

Consistency between studies

In a drug study containing 100 patients, a new cholesterol drug was found to decrease low-density lipoprotein (LDL) levels in 25% of the patients. In a second study containing 50 patients, the same drug administered at the same dosage was found to decrease LDL levels in 50% of the patients. Are the results of these two studies consistent with one another?

Even though in both studies 25 people (25% of 100 is 25 and 50% of 50 is 25) showed improvements in their LDL levels, the results of the studies are inconsistent. The results of the second study indicate that the drug has a much higher efficacy (desired result) than the results of the first study. Because 50 out of 150 total patients showed improvement on the medication, one could argue that the drug is effective in one-third (or approximately 33%) of patients. However, one should be wary of the reliability of results when they're not reproducible from one study to the next and when the sample size is fairly low.

Data organization

A nurse found the heart rates of eleven different patients to be 76, 80, 90, 86, 70, 76, 72, 88, 88, 68, and 88 beats per minutes. Organize this information in a table.

There are several ways to organize data in a table. Here is one example:

Patient Number	Heart Rate (bpm)
1	76
2	80
3	90
4	86
5	70
6	76
7	72
8	88
9	88
10	68
11	88

When making a table, be sure to label the columns appropriately.

Interpretation of graphs

<u>Example 1</u>
The following graph shows the ages of five patients a nurse is caring for in the hospital.

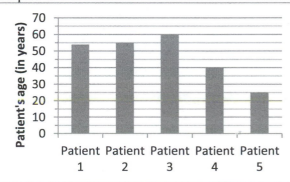

Use this graph to determine the age range of the patients for which the nurse is caring.

Use the graph to find the age of each patient: Patient 1 is 54 years old; Patient 2 is 55 years old; Patient 3 is 60 years old; Patient 4 is 40 years old; and Patient 5 is 25 years old. The age range is the age of the oldest patient minus the age of the youngest patient. In other words, 60 – 25 = 35. The age range is 35 years.

Example 2
Following is a line graph representing the heart rate of a patient during the day. Use the graph to answer the following questions:
The patient's minimum measured heart rate occurred at what time? The patient's maximum measured heart rate occurred at what time? At what times during the day did the patient have the same measured heart rate? What trends, if any, can you find about the patient's heart rate throughout the day?

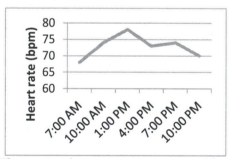

The patient's minimum measured heart rate occurred at the lowest data point on the graph, which is 68 bpm at 7:00 AM. The patient's maximum measured heart rate occurred at the highest data point on the graph, which is 78 bmp at 1:00 PM. The patient had the same measured heart rate of 74 bpm at 10:00 AM and 7:00 PM. The patient's heart rate increased through the morning to early afternoon, and generally declined as the afternoon progressed.

Independent and dependent variables

A patient told a doctor she feels fine that after running one mile but that her knee starts hurting after running two miles. Her knee throbs after running three miles and swells after running four. Identify the independent and dependent variables with regard to the distance she runs and her level of pain.

An independent variable is one that does not depend on any other variables in the situation. In this case, the distance the patient runs would be considered the independent variable. The dependent variable would be her level of pain because it depends on how far she runs.

Measurement

Measurement conversion

Convert the following measurements from the given unit of measurement to the unit measurement indicated:
1 foot = ___ yards
3 inches = ____ feet
5 inches = ____ centimeters
450 centimeters = _____ meters
32 ounces = ___ pounds
4 tons ___ pounds

1 foot = 1/3 yard
There are 12 inches in 1 foot, so 3 inches = 1/4 feet.
There are 2.54 centimeters in 1 inch, so 5 inches = 5(2.54) = 12.7 centimeters.
There are 100 centimeters in 1 meter, so 450 centimeters = 450/100 = 4.50 meters.
There are 16 ounces in 1 pound, so 32 ounces = 2 pounds.
There are 2,000 pounds in 1 ton, so 4 tons = 8,000 pounds.

Appropriate measurement unit

Determine the most appropriate
measurement unit given the situation:
 1: The volume of a tissue box: cubic
 inches, cubic feet, or square yards
 2: The area of a floor in a patient
 room: centimeters, square feet, or
 cubic meters
 3: The perimeter of an office building:
 inches, pounds, feet

To determine the appropriate unit of
measurement, first you must determine
what is being measured; for instance,
perimeter is measured in units, area in
square units, and volume in cubic units.
Next, you must determine the magnitude
of the measurements: for example, it
would make sense to measure the
distance between two cities in miles
rather than inches and the weight of a car
in tons rather than ounces.
 1: The volume of a tissue box is best
 measured in cubic inches.
 2: The area of a floor in patient room
 is best measured in square feet.
 3: The perimeter of an office building
 is best measured in feet.

Science

Human Body Science

Animal tissues

Animal tissues may be divided into seven categories:

- Epithelial - Tissue in which cells are joined together tightly. Skin tissue is an example.
- Connective - Connective tissue may be dense, loose or fatty. It protects and binds body parts.
- Cartilage - Cushions and provides structural support for body parts. It has a jelly-like base and is fibrous.
- Blood - Blood transports oxygen to cells and removes wastes. It also carries hormones and defends against disease.
- Bone - Bone is a hard tissue that supports and protects softer tissues and organs. Its marrow produces red blood cells.
- Muscle - Muscle tissue helps support and move the body. The three types of muscle tissue are smooth, cardiac, and skeletal.
- Nervous - Cells called neurons form a network through the body that control responses to changes in the external and internal environment. Some send signals to muscles and glands to trigger responses.

Integumentary system

The skin and its associated structures are called the integumentary system. It provides the following key functions:

- Protection of the body from abrasion and bacterial attack.
- Serves as a control mechanism for internal temperature.
- Provides a reserve of blood vessels that can be used as necessary.
- Produces vitamin D for metabolic purposes.

The covering of the skin is the epidermis and the layer beneath that is the dermis. The dermis consists of dense connective tissue which protects the body. Skin structure varies widely among animals according to the needs of the particular species. Pigments determine skin color. The process of keratinization results in a new layer of top skin in humans every month or so. This process helps the skin heal itself after minor injuries and forms a barrier against toxic substances and bacterial infections.

Skeletal system

The skeletal system has an important role in the following body functions:

- Movement - The action of skeletal muscles on bones moves the body.
- Mineral Storage - Bones serve as storage facilities for essential mineral ions.
- Support - Bones act as a framework and support system for the organs.
- Protection - Bones surround and protect key organs in the body.
- Blood Cell Formation - Red blood cells are produced in the marrow of certain bones.

Bones are classified as either long, short, flat, or irregular. They are a connective tissue with a base of pulp containing collagen and living cells. Red marrow, an important site of red blood cell production, fills the spongy tissue of many bones. Bone tissue is constantly regenerating itself as the mineral composition changes. This allows for special needs during growth periods and maintains calcium levels for the body.

Bone turnover can deteriorate in old age, particularly among women, leading to osteoporosis.

Skeletal system

The skeletal structure in humans contains both bones and cartilage. There are 206 bones in the human body, arranged in two parts:
- Axial skeleton - Includes the skull, sternum, ribs, and vertebral column (the spine).
- Appendicular skeleton - Includes the bones of the arms, feet, hands, legs, hips, and shoulders.

The flexible and curved backbone is supported by muscles and ligaments. Intervertebral discs are stacked one above another and provide cushioning for the backbone. Trauma or shock may cause these discs to herniate and cause pain. The sensitive spinal cord is enclosed in a cavity well protected by the bones of the vertebrae.

Joints are areas of contact adjacent to bones. Synovial joints are the most common, and are freely moveable. These may be found at the shoulders and knees. Cartilaginous joints fill the spaces between some bones and restrict movement. Examples of cartilaginous joints are those between vertebrae. Fibrous joints have fibrous tissue connecting bones and no cavity is present.

Muscular system

There are three types of muscle tissue: skeletal, cardiac, and smooth. There are over 600 muscles in the human body. All muscles have these three properties in common:
- Excitability - All muscle tissues have an electric gradient which can reverse when stimulated.
- Contraction - All muscle tissues have the ability to contract, or shorten.
- Elongate - Muscle tissues share the capacity to elongate, or relax.

Only skeletal muscle interacts with the skeleton to move the body. When they contract, the muscles transmit force to the attached bones. Working together, the muscles and bones act as a system of levers which move around the joints. A small contraction of a muscle can produce a large movement. A limb can be extended and rotated around a joint due to the way the muscles are arranged.

Digestive system

Most digestive systems function by the following means:
- Movement - Movement mixes and passes nutrients through the system and eliminates waste.
- Secretion - Enzymes, hormones, and other substances necessary for digestion are secreted into the digestive tract.
- Digestion - Includes the chemical breakdown of nutrients into smaller units that enter the internal environment.
- Absorption - The passage of nutrients through plasma membranes into the blood or lymph and then to the body.

The human digestive system consists of the mouth, pharynx, esophagus, stomach, small and large intestine, rectum, and anus. Enzymes and other secretions are infused into the digestive system to assist the absorption and processing of nutrients. The nervous and endocrine systems control the digestive system. Smooth muscle moves the food by peristalsis, contracting and relaxing to move nutrients along.

Mouth and stomach

Digestion begins in the mouth with the chewing and mixing of nutrients with saliva. Only humans and other mammals actually chew their food. Salivary glands are stimulated and secrete saliva. Saliva contains enzymes that initiate the breakdown of starch in digestion. Once swallowed, the food moves down the pharynx into the esophagus en route to the stomach.

The stomach is a flexible, muscular sac. It has three main functions:

- Mixing and storing food
- Dissolving and degrading food via secretions
- Controlling passage of food into the small intestine

Protein digestion begins in the stomach. Stomach acidity helps break down the food and make nutrients available for absorption. Smooth muscle contractions move nutrients into the small intestine where the absorption process begins.

Small intestine

In the digestive process, most nutrients are absorbed in the small intestine. Enzymes from the pancreas, liver, and stomach are transported to the small intestine to aid digestion. These enzymes act on fats, carbohydrates, nucleic acids, and proteins. Bile is a secretion of the liver and is particularly useful in breaking down fats. It is stored in the gall bladder between meals.

By the time food reaches the lining of the small intestine, it has been reduced to small molecules. The lining of the small intestine is covered with villi, tiny absorptive structures that greatly increase the surface area for interaction with chyme. Epithelial cells at the surface of the villi, called microvilli, further increase the ability of the small intestine to serve as the main absorption organ of the digestive tract.

Large intestine

Also called the colon, the large intestine concentrates, mixes, and stores waste material. A little over a meter in length, the colon ascends on the right side of the abdominal cavity, cuts across transversely to the left side, then descends and attaches to the rectum, a short tube for waste disposal.

When the rectal wall is distended by waste material, the nervous system triggers an impulse in the body to expel the waste from the rectum. A muscle sphincter at the end of the anus is stimulated to facilitate the expelling of waste matter.

The speed at which waste moves through the colon is influenced by the volume of fiber and other undigested material present. Without adequate bulk in the diet, it takes longer to move waste along, sometimes with negative effects. Lack of bulk in the diet has been linked to a number of disorders.

Circulatory system

The circulatory system is responsible for the internal transport of substances to and from the cells. The circulatory system usually consists of the following three parts:

- Blood - Blood is composed of water, solutes, and other elements in a fluid connective tissue.
- Blood Vessels - Tubules of different sizes that transport blood.
- Heart - The heart is a muscular pump providing the pressure necessary to keep blood flowing.

Circulatory systems can be either open or closed. Most animals have closed systems, where the heart and blood vessels are continually connected. As the blood moves through the system from larger tubules through smaller ones, the rate slows down. The flow of blood in the capillary beds, the smallest tubules, is quite slow.

A supplementary system, the lymph vascular system, cleans up excess fluids and proteins and returns them to the circulatory system.

Blood

Blood helps maintain a healthy internal environment in animals by carrying raw materials to cells and removing waste products. It helps stabilize internal pH and hosts various kinds of infection fighters.

An adult human has about five quarts of blood. Blood is composed of red and white blood cells, platelets, and plasma. Plasma constitutes over half of the blood volume. It is mostly water and serves as a solvent. Plasma contains plasma proteins, ions, glucose, amino acids, hormones, and dissolved gases.

Red blood cells transport oxygen to cells. Red blood cells form in the bone marrow and can live for about two months. These cells are constantly being replaced by fresh ones, keeping the total number relatively stable.

White blood cells defend the body against infection and remove various wastes. The types of white blood cells include lymphocytes, neutrophils, monocytes, eosinophils, and basophils.

Platelets are fragments of stem cells which serve an important function in blood clotting.

Heart

The heart is a muscular pump made of cardiac muscle tissue. It has four chambers; each half contains both an atrium and a ventricle, and the halves are separated by an AV valve. The valve is located between the ventricle and the artery leading away from the heart. Valves keep blood moving in a single direction and prevent any backwash into the chambers.

The heart has its own circulatory system with its own coronary arteries. The heart functions by contracting and relaxing. Atrial contraction fills the ventricles and ventricular contraction empties them, forcing circulation. This sequence is called the cardiac cycle. Cardiac muscles are attached to each other and signals for contractions spread rapidly. A complex electrical system controls the heartbeat as cardiac muscle cells produce and conduct electric signals. These muscles are said to be self-exciting, needing no external stimuli.

Blood pressure

Blood pressure is the fluid pressure generated by the cardiac cycle. Arterial blood pressure functions by transporting oxygen-poor blood into the lungs and oxygen-rich blood to the body tissues. Arteries branch into smaller arterioles which contract and expand based on signals from the body. Arterioles are the site where adjustments are made in blood delivery to specific areas based on complex communication from body systems.

Capillary beds are diffusion sites for exchanges between blood and interstitial fluid. A capillary has the thinnest wall of any blood vessel, consisting of a single layer of endothelial cells.

Capillaries merge into venues which in turn merge with larger diameter tubules called veins. Veins transport blood from body tissues back to the heart. Valves inside the veins facilitate this transport. The walls of veins are thin and contain smooth muscle and also function as blood volume reserves.

Lymphatic system

The main function of the lymphatic system is to return excess tissue fluid to the bloodstream. This system consists of transport vessels and lymphoid organs.

The lymph vascular system consists of lymph capillaries, lymph vessels, and lymph ducts. The major functions of the lymph vascular system are:

- The return of excess fluid to the blood.
- The return of protein from the capillaries.
- The transport of fats from the digestive tract.
- The disposal of debris and cellular waste.

Lymphoid organs include the lymph nodes, spleen, appendix, adenoids, thymus, tonsils, and small patches of tissue in the small intestine. Lymph nodes are located at intervals throughout the lymph vessel system. Each node contains lymphocytes and plasma cells. The spleen filters blood stores of red blood cells and macrophages. The thymus secretes hormones and is the major site of lymphocyte production.

Immune system

The body's general immune defenses include:

- Skin - An intact epidermis and dermis forms a formidable barrier against bacteria.
- Ciliated Mucous Membranes - Cilia sweep pathogens out of the respiratory tract.
- Glandular Secretions - Secretions from exocrine glands destroy bacteria.
- Gastric Secretions - Gastric acid destroys pathogens.
- Normal Bacterial Populations - Compete with pathogens in the gut and vagina.

In addition, phagocytes and inflammation responses mobilize white blood cells and chemical reactions to stop infection. These include localized redness, tissue repair, and fluid-seeping healing agents.

Additionally, plasma proteins act as the complement system to repel bacteria and pathogens.

Three types of white blood cells form the foundation of the body's immune system. They are:

- Macrophages - Phagocytes that alert T cells to the presence of foreign substances.
- T Lymphocytes - These directly attack cells infected by viruses and bacteria.
- B Lymphocytes - These cells target specific bacteria for destruction.

Memory cells, suppressor T cells, and helper T cells also contribute to the body's defense. Immune responses can be anti-body mediated when the response is to an antigen, or cell-mediated when the response is to already infected cells. These responses are controlled and measured counter-attacks that recede when the foreign agents are destroyed. Once an invader has attacked the body, if it returns it is immediately recognized and a secondary immune response occurs. This secondary response is rapid and powerful, much more so than the original response. These memory lymphocytes circulate throughout the body for years, alert to a possible new attack.

Nervous system

The human nervous system senses, interprets, and issues commands as a response to conditions in the body's environment. This process is made possible by a very complex communication system organized as a grid of neurons.
Messages are sent across the plasma membrane of neurons through a process called action potential. These messages occur when a neuron is stimulated past a

necessary threshold. These stimulations occur in a sequence from the stimulation point of one neuron to its contact with another neuron. At the point of contact, called a chemical synapse, a substance is released that stimulates or inhibits the action of the adjoining cell. This network fans out across the body and forms the framework for the nervous system. The direction the information flows depends on the specific organizations of nerve circuits and pathways.

Central nervous system

There are two primary components of the central nervous system:

- Spinal cord - The spinal cord is encased in the bony structure of the vertebrae, which protects and supports it. Its nervous tissue functions mainly with respect to limb movement and internal organ activity. Major nerve tracts ascend and descend from the spinal cord to the brain.
- Brain - The brain consists of the hindbrain, which includes the medulla oblongata, cerebellum, and pons. The midbrain integrates sensory signals and orchestrates responses to these signals. The forebrain includes the cerebrum, thalamus, and hypothalamus. The cerebral cortex is a thin layer of gray matter covering the cerebrum. The brain is divided into two hemispheres, with each responsible for multiple functions.

In addition, the peripheral nervous system consists of the nerves and ganglia throughout the body and includes sympathetic nerves which trigger the "fight or flight" response, and the parasympathetic nerves which control basic body function.

Respiration

Connected airways of the body (including the nasal cavities, pharynx, larynx, trachea, bronchi, and bronchioles) provide a transport highway for respiration. Alveoli at the end of this system serve as the gas exchange mechanism of the system.
As air is inhaled, oxygen brought into the lungs diffuses from the alveoli into pulmonary capillaries. It then diffuses into red blood cells and fuses with hemoglobin. When the oxygen-rich blood reaches the body tissues, the hemoglobin releases its oxygen, which diffuses out of the capillaries, through the interstitial fluid, and into the cells. The hemoglobin releases oxygen in response to body signals. Carbon dioxide then diffuses from cells, through interstitial fluid, into the bloodstream, completing the cycle.

Endocrine system

The endocrine system is responsible for secreting the hormones and other molecules that help regulate the entire body in both the short and the long term. There is a close working relationship between the endocrine system and the nervous system. The hypothalamus and the pituitary gland coordinate to serve as a neuroendrocrine control center. Hormone secretion is triggered by a variety of signals, including hormonal signs, chemical reactions, and environmental cues. Only cells with particular receptors can benefit from hormonal influence. This is the "key in the lock" model for hormonal action. Steroid hormones trigger gene activation and protein synthesis in some target cells. Protein hormones change the activity of existing enzymes in target cells. Hormones such as insulin work quickly when the body signals an urgent need. Slower acting hormones afford longer, gradual, and sometimes permanent changes in the body.

The eight major endocrine glands and their functions are:

- Adrenal cortex - Monitors blood sugar level; helps in lipid and protein metabolism.
- Adrenal medulla - Controls cardiac function; raises blood sugar and controls the size of blood vessels.
- Thyroid gland - Helps regulate metabolism and functions in growth and development.
- Parathyroid - Regulates calcium levels in the blood.
- Pancreas islets - Raises and lowers blood sugar; active in carbohydrate metabolism.
- Thymus gland - Plays a role in immune responses.
- Pineal gland - Has an influence on daily biorhythms and sexual activity.
- Pituitary gland - Plays an important role in growth and development.

Endocrine glands are intimately involved in a myriad of reactions, functions, and secretions that are crucial to the well-being of the body.

Animal reproduction

As a rule, animals produce sexually. Evolution has ensured that separation into male and female structures maximizes the chances for successful fertilization and nutritional support to the offspring. It has also played a role in shaping behaviors of animals to assure these goals.

Humans have a pair of primary reproductive organs, one for each gender: the sperm-producing testes in males and the egg-producing ovaries in females. These organs have supplementary ducts, glands, and supporting structures. Human males produce sperm continually from puberty onward. Females produce and release eggs on a monthly cycle. Hormones such as estrogen, progesterone, FSH, and LH control this cycle.

The six stages of development are gamete formation, fertilization, cleavage, gastrulation, organ formation, and the growth and development of specialized tissues. All tissues and organs arise from three germ layers: the endosperm, ectosperm, and mesoderm of the early embryo. Embryonic development requires the help of some embryonic membranes including the yolk sac, amnion, chorion, and allantois.

Demographic transition model

The demographic transition model is a representation of changes in population in industrial societies, created by demographer Warren Thompson. This model describes variations (transitions) in birth and death rates in developed nations over the past 200 years. The demographic transition model encompasses four transitional phases:

- Stage One is associated with pre-modern (that is, pre-industrialized) society; it characterizes most regions of the world through the 17th century. In this stage (the high stationary stage), birth and death rates are high and nearly equivalent, indicating that population growth is slow. The second stage in the demographic transition model is differentiated by a sharp increase in a society's population due to a dramatic decrease in the death rate. This transition occurred in the late 18th century in Western Europe and spread outward.
- Stage Two is associated with advances in public health such as the creation of food handling regulations and sewage disposal, as well as advances in agricultural

practices (including crop rotation) that helped to create a stable food source.

- Stage Three of the demographic transition model involves a decrease in a society's birth rate (following the rapid population growth in Stage Two). Most developed nations entered this phase late in the 19th century. Many hypotheses have been advanced to explain this phenomenon. For example, some have suggested that the decline in birth rates observed in developed societies is related to urbanization, which dilutes the high value traditionally placed on fertility; also, the costs attendant to urbanization make it less financially desirable for a family to have many children. The decline in birth rates has also been said to relate to medical advancements that decreased the rate of childhood mortality, or to improvements in contraceptive technology (though this occurred later, in the second half of the 20th century).
- In Stage Four of the demographic transition model, the populations of societies are either stable or declining. After the decline in birth rates, the general population grows older. If the fertility rate dips below replacement, the population experiences a rapid decline.

Important terms

- Birth rate: The birth rate of a society refers to the number of births per 1,000 people in that society. This figure, usually expressed as the crude birth rate (CBR), is calculated without

consideration of the sex or age of the population.
- Death rate: The death rate of a society is figured in the same manner but with regard to deaths rather than births and is expressed as the crude death rate (CDR).
- Fertility rate: The fertility rate of a society is the average number of children which would be born by a woman during her "childbearing" years. Replacement fertility is the fertility level at which women on the average are birthing just enough children to "replace" themselves and their partners in the population.
- Population momentum: Population momentum is the phenomenon whereby a society's population persists after the attainment of replacement fertility. This occurs at the end of Stage Three in the demographic transition model, due to the relatively high concentration of people of the same age in their "childbearing" years.

Life Science

Natural selection

Natural selection acts continually on an organism's phenotype and this activity affects the organism's genotype. Although there are multiple factors that affect gene pools, natural selection best explains the adaptations organisms make to survive in different environments. As Darwin recognized, natural selection is a key mechanism in evolution; it affects the phenotypes of microbes, plants, and animals over time and, in doing so, determines the way present day organisms look and behave. Major

- 43 -

considerations in the understanding of natural selection include the following topics:

- The concept of fitness.
- How genotypes are affected by phenotypes.
- The varieties of natural selection.
- The mechanisms of evolution.

Fitness

Geneticists have a specialized definition of fitness. They use the term to denote an organism's capacity to survive, mate, and reproduce. This ultimately equates to the probability or likelihood that the organism will be able to pass on its genetic information to the next generation. Fitness does not mean the strongest, biggest, and most dangerous individual. A more subtle combination of anatomy, physiology, biochemistry, and behavior are factors that determine genetic fitness.

Another way to understand genetic fitness is knowing that phenotypes affect survival and the ability to successfully reproduce. Phenotypes are genetically determined and genes contributing to fitness tend to increase over time.

Thus, the "fittest" organisms survive and pass on their genetic makeup to the next generation. This is what Darwin meant by "survival of the fittest," which is the cornerstone of Darwin's theory of evolution.

Influence of phenotype on genotype
Natural selection provides processes that tend to increase a population's adaptive abilities. The strongest phenotypes survive, prosper, and pass on their genetic code to the next generation. The new generation of phenotypes has a more fit genotype because they have inherited more adaptive characteristics. Thus, fitness thrives while the weak become extinct over time. This pattern, when repeated over many generations, develops strong, fit phenotypes that survive and reproduce offspring who are as fit or more fit than their parents. Sometimes this apparently inexorable movement can be modified by drastic external conditions such as wide variations in climate. It is important to remember that all extinct species were once fit and adapted to their environments. Unforeseen circumstances always have the potential to cause chaos in the physical world.

Selective processes

There are four major selective processes which may produce evolutionary change or preserve existing adaptive traits. They are:

- Normalizing or stabilizing selection simply protects and preserves a fit existing phenotype. This type of selection is strongest in environments that have remained stable for long periods of time. Examples include arid desert areas and Antarctic glaciers.
- Directional variation occurs when an environment favors a genetic variant which grows in frequency over a period of time.
- Disrupting or diversifying selection occurs when a population is confronted with extreme new conditions that are so diverse that no one phenotype can prosper without the expense of others. This selective process can lead to two or more phenotypes adapting to a different extreme condition of the environment.
- Balanced selection is when a heterozygote has a higher fitness level than either homozygote. This is also called hybrid

- 44 -

advantage, such as when mongrel dogs are heartier than purebred dogs.

Classification for living organisms

The main characteristic by which living organisms are classified is the degree to which they are related, not the degree to which they resemble each other. The science of classification is called taxonomy, a difficult science since the division lines between groups is not always clear. Some animals have characteristics of two separate groups.

The basic system of taxonomy involves placing an organism into a major kingdom (Moneran, Protist, Fungi, Plants, and Animals), and then dividing those kingdoms into phyla, then classes, then orders, then families, and finally genuses. For example, the family cat is in the kingdom of animals, the phylum of chordates, the class of mammals, the order of carnivores, the family of felidae, and the genus of felis. All species of living beings can be identified with Latin scientific names that are assigned by the worldwide binomial system. The genus name comes first, and is followed by the name of the species. The family cat is *felis domesticus*.

Although not part of taxonomy, behavior is also considered in identifying living beings. For example, birds are identified according to their songs or means of flight.

Passive transport mechanisms

Transport mechanisms allow for the movement of substances through membranes. Passive transport mechanisms include simple and facilitated diffusion and osmosis. They do not require energy from the cell. Diffusion is when particles are transported from areas of higher concentration to areas of lower concentration. When equilibrium is reached, diffusion stops. Examples are gas exchange (carbon dioxide and oxygen) during photosynthesis and the transport of oxygen from air to blood and from blood to tissue. Facilitated diffusion is when specific molecules are transported by a specific carrier protein. Carrier proteins vary in terms of size, shape, and charge. Glucose and amino acids are examples of substances transported by carrier proteins. Osmosis is the diffusion of water through a semi-permeable membrane from an area of higher concentration to one of lower concentration. Examples of osmosis include the absorption of water by plant roots and the alimentary canal. Plants lose and gain water through osmosis. A plant cell that swells because of water retention is said to be turgid.

Active transport mechanisms

Active transport mechanisms include exocytosis and endocytosis. Active transport involves transferring substances from areas of lower concentration to areas of higher concentration. Active transport requires energy in the form of ATP. Endocytosis is the ingestion of large particles into a cell, and can be categorized as phagocytosis (ingestion of a particle), pinocytosis (ingestion of a liquid), or receptor mediated. Endocytosis occurs when a substance is too large to cross a cell membrane. Endocytosis is a process by which eukaryotes ingest food particles. During phagocytosis, cell eating vesicles used during ingestion are quickly formed and unformed. Pinocytosis is also known as cell drinking. Exocytosis is the opposite of endocytosis. It is the expulsion or discharge of substances from a cell. A lysosome digests particles with enzymes, and can be expelled through exocytosis. A vacuole containing the substance to be expelled attaches to the cell membrane and expels the substance.

Cell

The cell is the basic organizational unit of all living things. Each piece within a cell has a function that helps organisms grow and survive. There are many different types of cells, but cells are unique to each type of organism. The one thing that all cells have in common is a membrane, which is comparable to a semi-permeable plastic bag. The membrane is composed of phospholipids. There are also some transport holes, which are proteins that help certain molecules and ions move in and out of the cell. The cell is filled with a fluid called cytoplasm or cytosol.

Within the cell are a variety of organelles, groups of complex molecules that help a cell survive, each with its own unique membrane that has a different chemical makeup from the cell membrane. The larger the cell, the more organelles it will need to live.

Cell cycle

The term cell cycle refers to the process by which a cell reproduces, which involves cell growth, the duplication of genetic material, and cell division. Complex organisms with many cells use the cell cycle to replace cells as they lose their functionality and wear out. The entire cell cycle in animal cells can take 24 hours. The time required varies among different cell types. Human skin cells, for example, are constantly reproducing. Some other cells only divide infrequently. Once neurons are mature, they do not grow or divide. The two ways that cells can reproduce are through meiosis and mitosis. When cells replicate through mitosis, the "daughter cell" is an exact replica of the parent cell. When cells divide through meiosis, the daughter cells have different genetic coding than the parent cell. Meiosis only happens in specialized reproductive cells called gametes.

Mitosis

The primary events that occur during mitosis are:

- Interphase: The cell prepares for division by replicating its genetic and cytoplasmic material. Interphase can be further divided into G_1, S, and G_2.
- Prophase: The chromatin thickens into chromosomes and the nuclear membrane begins to disintegrate. Pairs of centrioles move to opposite sides of the cell and spindle fibers begin to form. The mitotic spindle, formed from cytoskeleton parts, moves chromosomes around within the cell.
- Metaphase: The spindle moves to the center of the cell and chromosome pairs align along the center of the spindle structure.
- Anaphase: The pairs of chromosomes, called sisters, begin to pull apart, and may bend. When they are separated, they are called daughter chromosomes. Grooves appear in the cell membrane.
- Telophase: The spindle disintegrates, the nuclear membranes reform, and the chromosomes revert to chromatin. In animal cells, the membrane is pinched. In plant cells, a new cell wall begins to form.
- Cytokinesis: This is the physical splitting of the cell (including the cytoplasm) into two cells. Some believe this occurs following telophase. Others say it occurs from anaphase, as the cell begins to furrow, through telophase, when the cell actually splits into two.

Meiosis

Meiosis has the same phases as mitosis, but they happen twice. In addition, different events occur during some phases of meiosis than mitosis. The events that occur during the first phase of meiosis are interphase (I), prophase (I), metaphase (I), anaphase (I), telophase (I), and cytokinesis (I). During this first phase of meiosis, chromosomes cross over, genetic material is exchanged, and tetrads of four chromatids are formed. The nuclear membrane dissolves. Homologous pairs of chromatids are separated and travel to different poles. At this point, there has been one cell division resulting in two cells. Each cell goes through a second cell division, which consists of prophase (II), metaphase (II), anaphase (II), telophase (II), and cytokinesis (II). The result is four daughter cells with different sets of chromosomes. The daughter cells are haploid, which means they contain half the genetic material of the parent cell. The second phase of meiosis is similar to the process of mitosis. Meiosis encourages genetic diversity.

Photosynthesis

Photosynthesis is the conversion of sunlight into energy in plant cells, and also occurs in some types of bacteria and protists. Carbon dioxide and water are converted into glucose during photosynthesis, and light is required during this process. Cyanobacteria are thought to be the descendants of the first organisms to use photosynthesis about 3.5 billion years ago. Photosynthesis is a form of cellular respiration. It occurs in chloroplasts that use thylakoids, which are structures in the membrane that contain light reaction chemicals. Chlorophyll is a pigment that absorbs light. During the process, water is used and oxygen is released. The equation for the chemical reaction that occurs during photosynthesis is $6H_2O + 6CO_2 \rightarrow C_6H_{12}O_6 + 6O_2$. During photosynthesis, six molecules of water and six molecules of carbon dioxide react to form one molecule of sugar and six molecules of oxygen.

Cellular respiration

Cellular respiration refers to a set of metabolic reactions that convert chemical bonds into energy stored in the form of ATP. Respiration includes many oxidation and reduction reactions that occur thanks to the electron transport system within the cell. Oxidation is a loss of electrons and reduction is a gain of electrons. Electrons in C-H (carbon/hydrogen) and C-C (carbon/carbon) bonds are donated to oxygen atoms. Processes involved in cellular respiration include glycolysis, the Krebs cycle, the electron transport chain, and chemiosmosis. The two forms of respiration are aerobic and anaerobic. Aerobic respiration is very common, and oxygen is the final electron acceptor. In anaerobic respiration, the final electron acceptor is not oxygen. Aerobic respiration results in more ATP than anaerobic respiration. Fermentation is another process by which energy is converted.

DNA

Chromosomes consist of genes, which are single units of genetic information. Genes are made up of deoxyribonucleic acid (DNA). DNA is a nucleic acid located in the cell nucleus. There is also DNA in the mitochondria. DNA replicates to pass on genetic information. The DNA in almost all cells is the same. It is also involved in the biosynthesis of proteins. The model or structure of DNA is described as a double helix. A helix is a curve, and a double helix is two congruent curves connected by horizontal members. The model can be likened to a spiral staircase. It is right-handed. The British scientist Rosalind

- 47 -

Elsie Franklin is credited with taking the x-ray diffraction image in 1952 that was used by Francis Crick and James Watson to formulate the double-helix model of DNA and speculate about its important role in carrying and transferring genetic information.

Structure

DNA has a double helix shape, resembles a twisted ladder, and is compact. It consists of nucleotides. Nucleotides consist of a five-carbon sugar (pentose), a phosphate group, and a nitrogenous base. Two bases pair up to form the rungs of the ladder. The "side rails" or backbone consists of the covalently bonded sugar and phosphate. The bases are attached to each other with hydrogen bonds, which are easily dismantled so replication can occur. Each base is attached to a phosphate and to a sugar. There are four types of nitrogenous bases: adenine (A), guanine (G), cytosine (C), and thymine (T). There are about 3 billion bases in human DNA. The bases are mostly the same in everybody, but their order is different. It is the order of these bases that creates diversity in people. Adenine (A) pairs with thymine (T), and cytosine (C) pairs with guanine (G).

Replication

Pairs of chromosomes are composed of DNA, which is tightly wound to conserve space. When replication starts, it unwinds. The steps in DNA replication are controlled by enzymes. The enzyme helicase instigates the deforming of hydrogen bonds between the bases to split the two strands. The splitting starts at the A-T bases (adenine and thymine) as there are only two hydrogen bonds. The cytosine-guanine base pair has three bonds. The term "origin of replication" is used to refer to where the splitting starts. The portion of the DNA that is unwound to be replicated is called the replication fork. Each strand of DNA is transcribed by an mRNA. It copies the DNA onto itself, base by base, in a complementary manner. The exception is that uracil replaces thymine.

RNA and DNA

RNA and DNA differ in terms of structure and function. RNA has a different sugar than DNA. It has ribose rather than deoxyribose sugar. The RNA nitrogenous bases are adenine (A), guanine (G), cytosine (C), and uracil (U). Uracil is found only in RNA and thymine in found only in DNA. RNA consists of a single strand and DNA has two strands. If straightened out, DNA has two side rails. RNA only has one "backbone," or strand of sugar and phosphate group components. RNA uses the fully hydroxylated sugar pentose, which includes an extra oxygen compared to deoxyribose, which is the sugar used by DNA. RNA supports the functions carried out by DNA. It aids in gene expression, replication, and transportation.

RNA

RNA acts as a helper to DNA and carries out a number of other functions. Types of RNA include ribosomal RNA (rRNA), transfer RNA (tRNA), and messenger RNA (mRNA). Viruses can use RNA to carry their genetic material to DNA. Ribosomal RNA is not believed to have changed much over time. For this reason, it can be used to study relationships in organisms. Messenger RNA carries a copy of a strand of DNA and transports it from the nucleus to the cytoplasm. Transcription is the process whereby DNA uses RNA in transcription. DNA unwinds itself and serves as a template while RNA is being assembled. The DNA molecules are copied to RNA. Translation is the process whereby ribosomes use transcribed RNA to put together the needed protein. Transfer RNA is a molecule that helps in the translation process, and is found in the cytoplasm. Ribosomal RNA is in the ribosomes.

Mutations

Gene disorders are the result of DNA mutations. DNA mutations lead to unfavorable gene disorders, but also provide genetic variability. This diversity can lead to increased survivability of a species. Mutations can be neutral, beneficial, or harmful. Mutations can be hereditary, meaning they are passed from parent to child. Polymorphism refers to differences in humans, such as eye and hair color, that may have originally been the result of gene mutations, but are now part of the normal variation of the species. Mutations can be de novo, meaning they happen either only in sex cells or shortly after fertilization. They can also be acquired, or somatic. These are the kinds that happen as a result of DNA changes due to environmental factors or replication errors. Mosaicism is when a mutation happens in a cell during an early embryonic stage. The result is that some cells will have the mutation and some will not.

DNA mutation

A DNA mutation occurs when the normal gene sequence is altered. Mutations can happen when DNA is damaged as a result of environmental factors, such as chemicals, radiation, or ultraviolet rays from the sun. It can also happen when errors are made during DNA replication. The phosphate-sugar side rail of DNA can be damaged if the bonds between oxygen and phosphate groups are disassociated. Translocation happens when the broken bonds attempt to bond with other DNA. This repair can cause a mutation. The nucleotide itself can be altered. A C, for example, might look like a T. During replication, the damaged C is replicated as a T and paired with a G, which is incorrect base pairing. Another way mutations can occur is if an error is made by the DNA polymerase while replicating a base. This happens about once for every 100,000,000 bases. A repair protein proofreads the code, however, so the mistake is usually repaired.

Gene, genotype, phenotype, and allele

A gene is a portion of DNA that identifies how traits are expressed and passed on in an organism. A gene is part of the genetic code. Collectively, all genes form the genotype of an individual. The genotype includes genes that may not be expressed, such as recessive genes. The phenotype is the physical, visual manifestation of genes. It is determined by the basic genetic information and how genes have been affected by their environment. An allele is a variation of a gene. Also known as a trait, it determines the manifestation of a gene. This manifestation results in a specific physical appearance of some facet of an organism, such as eye color or height. For example the genetic information for eye color is a gene. The gene variations responsible for blue, green, brown, or black eyes are called alleles. Locus (pl. loci) refers to the location of a gene or alleles.

Dominant and recessive

Gene traits are represented in pairs with an upper case letter for the dominant trait (A) and a lower case letter for the recessive trait (a). Genes occur in pairs (AA, Aa, or aa). There is one gene on each chromosome half supplied by each parent organism. Since half the genetic material is from each parent, the offspring's traits are represented as a combination of these. A dominant trait only requires one gene of a gene pair for it to be expressed in a phenotype, whereas a recessive requires both genes in order to be manifested. For example, if the mother's genotype is Dd and the father's is dd, the possible combinations are Dd and dd. The

- 49 -

dominant trait will be manifested if the genotype is DD or Dd. The recessive trait will be manifested if the genotype is dd. Both DD and dd are homozygous pairs. Dd is heterozygous.

Monohybrid and hybrid crosses

Genetic crosses are the possible combinations of alleles, and can be represented using Punnett squares. A monohybrid cross refers to a cross involving only one trait. Typically, the ratio is 3:1 (DD, Dd, Dd, dd), which is the ratio of dominant gene manifestation to recessive gene manifestation. This ratio occurs when both parents have a pair of dominant and recessive genes. If one parent has a pair of dominant genes (DD) and the other has a pair of recessive (dd) genes, the recessive trait cannot be expressed in the next generation because the resulting crosses all have the Dd genotype. A dihybrid cross refers to one involving more than one trait, which means more combinations are possible. The ratio of genotypes for a dihybrid cross is 9:3:3:1 when the traits are not linked. The ratio for incomplete dominance is 1:3:1:, which corresponds to dominant, mixed, and recessive phenotypes.

Mendel's laws and Punnett squares

Mendel's laws are the law of segregation (the first law) and the law of independent assortment (the second law). The law of segregation states that there are two alleles and that half of the total number of alleles are contributed by each parent organism. The law of independent assortment states that traits are passed on randomly and are not influenced by other traits. The exception to this is linked traits. A Punnett square can illustrate how alleles combine from the contributing genes to form various phenotypes. One set of a parent's genes are put in columns, while the genes from the other parent are placed in rows. The allele combinations are shown in each cell. When two different alleles are present in a pair, the dominant one is expressed. A Punnett square can be used to predict the outcome of crosses.

Important terms

- Nucleus (pl. nuclei): This is a small structure that contains the chromosomes and regulates the DNA of a cell. The nucleus is the defining structure of eukaryotic cells, and all eukaryotic cells have a nucleus. The nucleus is responsible for the passing on of genetic traits between generations. The nucleus contains a nuclear envelope, nucleoplasm, a nucleolus, nuclear pores, chromatin, and ribosomes.
- Chromosomes: These are highly condensed, threadlike rods of DNA. Short for deoxyribonucleic acid, DNA is the genetic material that stores information about the plant or animal.
- Chromatin: This consists of the DNA and protein that make up chromosomes.
- Nucleolus (nucleole): This structure contained within the nucleus consists of protein. It is small, round, does not have a membrane, is involved in protein synthesis, and synthesizes and stores RNA (ribonucleic acid).
- Nuclear envelope: This encloses the structures of the nucleus. It consists of inner and outer membranes made of lipids.
- Nuclear pores: These are involved in the exchange of material between the nucleus and the cytoplasm.
- Nucleoplasm: This is the liquid within the nucleus, and is similar to cytoplasm.

- Cytosol: This is the liquid material in the cell. It is mostly water, but also contains some floating molecules.
- Cytoplasm: This is a general term that refers to cytosol and the substructures (organelles) found within the plasma membrane, but not within the nucleus.
- Cell membrane (plasma membrane): This defines the cell by acting as a barrier. It helps keeps cytoplasm in and substances located outside the cell out. It also determines what is allowed to enter and exit the cell.
- Endoplasmic reticulum: The two types of endoplasmic reticulum are rough (has ribosomes on the surface) and smooth (does not have ribosomes on the surface). It is a tubular network that comprises the transport system of a cell. It is fused to the nuclear membrane and extends through the cytoplasm to the cell membrane.
- Mitochondrion (pl. mitochondria): These cell structures vary in terms of size and quantity. Some cells may have one mitochondrion, while others have thousands. This structure performs various functions such as generating ATP, and is also involved in cell growth and death. Mitochondria contain their own DNA that is separate from that contained in the nucleus.
- Ribosomes: Ribosomes are involved in synthesizing proteins from amino acids. They are numerous, making up about one quarter of the cell. Some cells contain thousands of ribosome. Some are mobile and some are embedded in the rough endoplasmic reticulum.
- Golgi complex (Golgi apparatus): This is involved in synthesizing materials such as proteins that are transported out of the cell. It is located near the nucleus and consists of layers of membranes.
- Vacuoles: These are sacs used for storage, digestion, and waste removal. There is one large vacuole in plant cells. Animal cells have small, sometimes numerous vacuoles.
- Vesicle: This is a small organelle within a cell. It has a membrane and performs varying functions, including moving materials within a cell.
- Cytoskeleton: This consists of microtubules that help shape and support the cell.
- Microtubules: These are part of the cytoskeleton and help support the cell. They are made of protein.
- Centrosome: This is comprised of the pair of centrioles located at right angles to each other and surrounded by protein. The centrosome is involved in mitosis and the cell cycle.
- Centriole: These are cylinder-shaped structures near the nucleus that are involved in cellular division. Each cylinder consists of nine groups of three microtubules. Centrioles occur in pairs.
- Lysosome: This digests proteins, lipids, and carbohydrates, and also transports undigested substances to the cell membrane so they can be removed. The shape of a lysosome depends on the material being transported.
- Cilia (singular: cilium): These are appendages extending from the surface of the cell, the movement of which causes the cell to move. They can also result in fluid being moved by the cell.

- Flagella: These are tail-like structures on cells that use whip-like movements to help the cell move. They are similar to cilia, but are usually longer and not as numerous. A cell usually only has one or a few flagella.
- Cell wall: Made of cellulose and composed of numerous layers, the cell wall provides plants with a sturdy barrier that can hold fluid within the cell. The cell wall surrounds the cell membrane.
- Chloroplast: This is a specialized organelle that plant cells use for photosynthesis, which is the process plants use to create food energy from sunlight. Chloroplasts contain chlorophyll, which has a green color.
- Plastid: This is a membrane-bound organelle found in plant cells that is used to make chemical compounds and store food. It can also contain pigments used during photosynthesis. Plastids can develop into more specialized structures such as chloroplasts, chromoplasts (make and hold yellow and orange pigments), amyloplasts (store starch), and leucoplasts (lack pigments, but can become differentiated).
- Plasmodesmata (sing. plasmodesma): These are channels between the cell walls of plant cells that allow for transport between cells.
- Lipid: Lipids take many forms and have varying functions, such as storing energy and acting as a building block of cell membranes. Lipids are produced by anabolysis.
- Organelle: This is a general term that refers to an organ or smaller structure within a cell. Membrane-bound organelles are found in eukaryotic cells.

- RNA: RNA is short for ribonucleic acid, which is a type of molecule that consists of a long chain (polymer) of nucleotide units.
- Polymer: This is a compound of large molecules formed by repeating monomers.
- Monomer: A monomer is a small molecule. It is a single compound that forms chemical bonds with other monomers to make a polymer.
- Nucleotides: These are molecules that combine to form DNA and RNA. They can be easily stained to make them more visible.
- Nucleoid: This is the nucleus-like, irregularly-shaped mass of DNA that contains the chromatin in a prokaryotic cell.

Earth and Physical Science

Proton, electron, and neutron

The three most important subatomic particles are the proton, electron, and neutron. Protons are the positively charged particles in the nucleus, with a mass of 1.67252×10^{-24} g. This is approximately 1,840 times the mass of the oppositely charged electron, 9.1095×10^{-28} g. Neutrons are also present in the nucleus, are electrically neutral, and have a mass slightly greater than that of protons, 1.67497×10^{-24} g. The electrons are attracted to the positively charged nucleus by the electrostatic or Coulomb force, which is directly proportional to the charge of the nucleus and inversely proportional to the square of the distance from the nucleus. The protons and neutrons are held together in the nucleus by the strong nuclear force. This nuclear force is known to be much stronger than the electrostatic force since the protons do not repel one another.

Atomic number, atomic mass number, and isotope

All atoms can be identified by the number of protons and neutrons that they contain. The atomic number, often denoted as Z, is the number of protons in the nucleus of each atom of an element. In an electrically neutral atom, the number of protons is equal to the number of electrons. The atomic mass number, often denoted as A, is the total number of nucleons (neutrons and protons present in the nucleus) in each atom of an element. Atoms that have the same atomic number but different mass numbers are called isotopes. A similar term is nuclide, which refers to an atom with a given number of protons and neutrons. Atoms of a given element typically do not all have the same mass. For example, there are three hydrogen isotopes: protium, which has one proton and no neutrons; deuterium, which has one proton and one neutron; and tritium, which has one proton and two neutrons. Isotopes are denoted by the element symbol, preceded in superscript and subscript by the mass number and atomic number, respectively. For instance, the notations for protium, deuterium, and tritium are, respectively:

$$^1_1H, ^2_1H, \text{ and } ^3_1H.$$

Matter

Matter is defined as anything that occupies space and has mass. Categories of matter include atoms, elements, molecules, compounds, substances and mixtures:

- An atom is the basic unit of an element that can enter into a chemical reaction.
- An element is a substance that cannot be separated into simpler substances by chemical means.
- A molecule is the smallest division of a compound that can exist in a natural state.
- A compound is a substance composed of atoms of two or more elements chemically united in fixed proportions.
- A substance is a form of matter that has a definite or constant composition and distinct properties.
- A mixture is a combination of two or more substances in which the substances retain their unique identities.

Organization of matter

An element is the most basic type of matter. It has unique properties and cannot be broken down into other elements. The smallest unit of an element is the atom. A chemical combination of two or more types of elements is called a compound. Compounds often have properties that are very different from those of their constituent elements. The smallest independent unit of an element or compound is known as a molecule. Most elements are found somewhere in nature in single-atom form, but a few elements only exist naturally in pairs. These are called diatomic elements, of which some of the most common are hydrogen, nitrogen, and oxygen. Elements and compounds are represented by chemical symbols, one or two letters, most often the first in the element name. More than one atom of the same element in a compound is represented with a subscript number designating how many atoms of that element are present. Water, for instance, contains two hydrogens and one oxygen. Thus, the chemical formula is H_2O. Methane contains one carbon and four hydrogens, so its formula is CH_4.

- 53 -

States of matter

The three states in which matter can exist are solid, liquid, and gas. They differ from each other in the motion of and attraction between individual molecules. In a solid, the molecules have little or no motion and are heavily attracted to neighboring molecules, giving them a definite structure. This structure may be ordered/crystalline or random/amorphous. Liquids also have considerable attraction between molecules, but the molecules are much more mobile, having no set structure. In a gas, the molecules have little or no attraction to one another and are constantly in motion. They are separated by distances that are very large in comparison to the size of the molecules. Gases easily expand to fill whatever space is available. Unlike solids and liquids, gases are easily compressible.

The three states of matter can be traversed by the addition or removal of heat. For example, when a solid is heated to its melting point, it can begin to form a liquid. However, in order to transition from solid to liquid, additional heat must be added at the melting point to overcome the latent heat of fusion. Upon further heating to its boiling point, the liquid can begin to form a gas, but again, additional heat must be added at the boiling point to overcome the latent heat of vaporization.

In the solid state, water is less dense than in the liquid state. This can be observed quite simply by noting that an ice cube floats at the surface of a glass of water. Were this not the case, ice would not form on the surface of lakes and rivers in those regions of the world where the climate produces temperatures below the freezing point. If water behaved as other substances, lakes and rivers would freeze from the bottom up and be detrimental to many forms of aquatic life. The lower density of ice occurs because of a combination of the unique structure of the water molecule and hydrogen bonding. In the case of ice, each oxygen atom is bound to four hydrogen atoms, two covalently and two by hydrogen bonds. This forms an ordered, roughly tetrahedral structure that prevents the molecules from getting close to each other. As such, there are empty spaces in the structure that account for the low density of ice.

Physical and chemical properties of matter

If a property of a substance can be observed and measured without change it is a physical property. Density, melting point and boiling point are examples of physical properties.

If a chemical change must be carried out in order to observe and measure a property, then the property is a chemical property. For example, when hydrogen gas is burned in oxygen, it forms water. This is a chemical property of hydrogen because after burning a different chemical substance – water – is all that remains. The hydrogen cannot be recovered from the water by means of a physical change such as freezing or boiling.

The table below outlines the characteristic properties of the three states of matter:

- 54 -

State of matter	Volume/ shape	Density	Compressibility	Molecular motion
Gas	Assumes volume and shape of its container	Low	High	Very free motion
Liquid	Volume remains constant but it assumes shape of its container	High	Slightly	Move past each other freely
Solid	Definite volume and shape	High	Incompressible	Vibrates around fixed positions

Types of Phase change

A substance that is undergoing a change from a solid to a liquid is said to be melting. If this change occurs in the opposite direction, from liquid to solid, this change is called freezing. A liquid which is being converted to a gas is undergoing vaporization. The reverse of this process is known as condensation. Direct transitions from gas to solid and solid to gas are much less common in everyday life, but they can occur given the proper conditions. Solid to gas conversion is known as sublimation, while the reverse is called deposition.

Evaporation: Evaporation is the change of state in a substance from a liquid to a gaseous form at a temperature below its boiling point (the temperature at which all of the molecules in a liquid are changed to gas through vaporization). Some of the molecules at the surface of a liquid always maintain enough heat energy to escape the cohesive forces exerted on them by neighboring molecules. At higher temperatures, the molecules in a substance move more rapidly, increasing their number with enough energy to break out of the liquid

form. The rate of evaporation is higher when more of the surface area of a liquid is exposed (as in a large water body, such as an ocean). The amount of moisture already in the air also affects the rate of evaporation—if there is a significant amount of water vapor in the air around a liquid, some evaporated molecules will return to the liquid. The speed of the evaporation process is also decreased by increased atmospheric pressure.

Condensation: Condensation is the phase change in a substance from a gaseous to liquid form; it is the opposite of evaporation or vaporization. When temperatures decrease in a gas, such as water vapor, the material's component molecules move more slowly. The decreased motion of the molecules enables intermolecular cohesive forces to pull the molecules closer together and, in water, establish hydrogen bonds. Condensation can also be caused by an increase in the pressure exerted on a gas, which results in a decrease in the substance's volume (it reduces the distance between particles). In the hydrologic cycle, this process is initiated when warm air containing water vapor rises and then cools. This occurs due to convection in the air, meteorological fronts, or lifting over high land formations.

Formation of molecules

Electrons in an atom can orbit different levels around the nucleus. They can absorb or release energy, which can change the location of their orbit or even allow them to break free from the atom. The outermost layer is the valence layer, which contains the valence electrons. The valence layer tends to have or share eight electrons. Molecules are formed by a chemical bond between atoms, a bond which occurs at the valence level. Two basic types of bonds are covalent and ionic. A covalent bond is formed when atoms share electrons. An ionic bond is formed when an atom transfers an electron to another atom. A hydrogen bond is a weak bond between a hydrogen atom of one molecule and an electronegative atom (such as nitrogen, oxygen, or fluorine) of another molecule. The Van der Waals force is a weak force between molecules. This type of force is much weaker than actual chemical bonds between atoms.

Interaction of atoms to form compounds

Atoms interact by transferring or sharing the electrons furthest from the nucleus. Known as the outer or valence electrons, they are responsible for the chemical properties of an element. Bonds between atoms are created when electrons are paired up by being transferred or shared. If electrons are transferred from one atom to another, the bond is ionic. If electrons are shared, the bond is covalent. Atoms of the same element may bond together to form molecules or crystalline solids. When two or more different types of atoms bind together chemically, a compound is made. The physical properties of compounds reflect the nature of the interactions among their molecules. These interactions are determined by the structure of the molecule, including the atoms they consist of and the distances and angles between them.

Chemical bonds between atoms

A union between the electron structures of atoms is called chemical bonding. An atom may gain, surrender, or share its electrons with another atom it bonds with. Listed below are three types of chemical bonding.

- Ionic bonding - When an atom gains or loses electrons it becomes positively or negatively charged, turning it into an ion. An ionic bond is a relationship between two oppositely charged ions.
- Covalent bonding - Atoms that share electrons have what is called a covalent bond. Electrons shared equally have a non-polar bond, while electrons shared unequally have a polar bond.
- Hydrogen bonding - The atom of a molecule interacts with a hydrogen atom in the same area. Hydrogen bonds can also form between two different parts of the same molecule, as in the structure of DNA and other large molecules.

Ionic bonding
The transfer of electrons from one atom to another is called ionic bonding. Atoms that lose or gain electrons are referred to as ions. The gain or loss of electrons will result in an ion having a positive or negative charge.
Here is an example:
Take an atom of sodium (Na) and an atom of chlorine (Cl). The sodium atom has a total of 11 electrons as well as one electron in its outer shell. The chlorine

has 17 electrons as well as 7 electrons in its outer shell. From this, the atomic number, or number of protons, of sodium can be calculated as 11 because the number of protons equals the number of electrons in an atom. When sodium chloride (NaCl) is formed, one electron from sodium transfers to chlorine. Ions have charges. They are written with a plus (+) or minus (-) symbol. Ions in a compound are attracted to each other because they have opposite charges.

Covalent bonding

Covalent bonding is characterized by the sharing of one or more pairs of electrons between two atoms or between an atom and another covalent bond. This produces an attraction to repulsion stability that holds these molecules together. Atoms have the tendency to share electrons with each other so that all outer electron shells are filled. The resultant bonds are always stronger than the intermolecular hydrogen bond and are similar in strength to ionic bonds. Covalent bonding occurs most frequently between atoms with similar electronegativities. Nonmetals are more likely to form covalent bonds than metals since it is more difficult for nonmetals to liberate an electron, electron sharing takes place when one species encountered another species with similar electronegativity. Covalent bonding of metals is important in both process chemistry and industrial catalysis.

Periodicity

Periodicity describes the predictable and incremental nature of elements' properties and places them on the periodic table accordingly. An atom of every element has unique properties such as number of electrons, density, and mass. The periodic table is arranged such that elements near each other are more alike in these properties than those that are far apart on the table. Periodicity enables the prediction of properties and atomic configurations based on known trends represented by the position of elements on the table. One such trend is the number of electrons; reading from left to right on any given row of the table, each element contains one more electron than the one immediately preceding it. On row 4, for example, K contains 19 electrons and the next element, Ca, contains 20.

Periodic table

The periodic table is a tabular arrangement of the elements and is organized according to periodic law. The properties of the elements depend on their atomic structure and vary with atomic number. It shows periodic trends of physical and chemical properties and identifies families of elements with similar properties. In the periodic table, the elements are arranged by atomic number in horizontal rows called periods and vertical columns called groups or families. They are further categorized as metals, metalloids, or nonmetals. The majority of known elements are metals; there are seventeen nonmetals and eight metalloids. Metals are situated at the left end of the periodic table, nonmetals to the right and metalloids between the two.

Most periodic tables contain the element's atomic weight, number, and symbol in each box. The position of an element in the table reveals its group, its block, and whether it is a representative, transition, or inner transition element. Its position also shows the element as a metal, nonmetal, or metalloid. For the representative elements, the last digit of the group number reveals the number of outer-level electrons. Roman numerals for the A groups also reveal the number of outer level electrons within the group. The position of the element in the table reveals its electronic configuration and how it differs in atomic size from neighbors in its period or group. In this example, Boron has an atomic number of 5 and an atomic weight of 10.811. It is found in group 13, in which all atoms of the group have 3 valence electrons; the group's Roman numeral representation is IIIA.

Important features and structure
The most important feature of the table is its arrangement according to periodicity, or the predictable trends observable in atoms. The arrangement enables classification, organization, and prediction of important elemental properties. The table is organized in horizontal rows called Periods, and vertical columns called Groups or Families. Groups of elements share predictable characteristics, the most important of which is that their outer energy levels have the same configuration of electrons. For example, the highest group is group 18, the noble gases. Each element in this group has a full complement of electrons in its outer level, making the reactivity low. Elements in periods also share some common properties, but most classifications rely more heavily on groups. A typical periodic table shows the elements' symbols and atomic number, the number of protons in the atomic nucleus. Some more detailed tables also list atomic mass, electronegativity, and other data.

Chemical reactivity
Reactivity refers to the tendency of a substance to engage in chemical reactions. If that tendency is high, the substance is said to be highly reactive, or to have high reactivity. Because the basis of a chemical reaction is the transfer of electrons, reactivity depends upon the presence of uncommitted electrons which are available for transfer. Periodicity allows us to predict an element's reactivity based on its position on the periodic table. High numbered groups on the right side of the table have a fuller complement of electrons in their outer

levels, making them less likely to react. Noble gases, on the far right of the table, each have eight electrons in the outer level, with the exception of He, which has two. Because atoms tend to lose or gain electrons to reach an ideal of eight in the outer level, these elements have very low reactivity.

Groups and periods in terms of reactivity
Reading left to right within a period, each element contains one more electron than the one preceding it. (Note that H and He are in the same period, though nothing is between them and they are in different groups.) As electrons are added, their attraction to the nucleus increases, meaning that as we read to the right in a period, each atom's electrons are more densely compacted, more strongly bound to the nucleus, and less likely to be pulled away in reactions. As we read down a group, each successive atom's outer electrons are less tightly bound to the nucleus, thus increasing their reactivity, because the principal energy levels are increasingly full as we move downward within the group. Principal energy levels shield the outer energy levels from nuclear attraction, allowing the valence electrons to react. For this reason, noble gases farther down the group can react under certain circumstances.

Chemical reactions

The classic chemical reaction is a transfer of electrons resulting in a transformation of the substances involved in the reaction. The changes may be in composition or configuration of a compound or substance, and result in one or more products being generated which were not present in isolation before the reaction occurred. For instance, when oxygen reacts with methane (CH_4), water and carbon dioxide are the products; one set of substances ($CH_4 + O$) was transformed into a new set of substances ($CO_2 + H_2O$). Reactions are classified in many ways, some of which are as follows: as combination or synthesis, in which two or more compounds unite to form a more complex compound; decomposition, in which a compound is broken down into its constituent compounds or elements; and isomerization, in which compounds undergo structural changes without changing their atomic composition.

Chemical reactions measured in human time can take place quickly or slowly. They can take fractions of a second or billions of years. The rates of chemical reactions are determined by how frequently reacting atoms and molecules interact. Rates are also influenced by the temperature and various properties (such as shape) of the reacting materials. Catalysts accelerate chemical reactions, while inhibitors decrease reaction rates. Some types of reactions release energy in the form of heat and light. Some types of reactions involve the transfer of either electrons or hydrogen ions between reacting ions, molecules, or atoms. In other reactions, chemical bonds are broken down by heat or light to form reactive radicals with electrons that will readily form new bonds. Processes such as the formation of ozone and greenhouse gases in the atmosphere and the burning and processing of fossil fuels are controlled by radical reactions.

Basic mechanisms
Chemical reactions normally occur when electrons are transferred from one atom or molecule to another. Reactions and reactivity depend on the octet rule, which describes the tendency of atoms to gain or lose electrons until their outer energy levels contain eight. Reactions always result in a change in composition or constitution of a compound. They depend on the presence of a reactant, or substance undergoing change, a reagent, or partner in the reaction less transformed than the reactant (such as a catalyst), and products, or the final result

of the reaction. Reaction conditions, or environmental factors, are also important components in reactions. These include conditions such as temperature, pressure, concentration, whether the reaction occurs in solution, the type of solution, and presence or absence of catalysts. Reactions are described with the following equation:

$$\text{Reagent(s)} \quad \text{Reactant(s)} \quad \rightarrow \quad \text{Product(s)} \quad \text{Reaction conditions}$$

Exothermic, endothermic, activation energy, and reaction equilibrium
Exothermic reactions are chemical reactions in which energy is released or produced, such as in combustion. In endothermic reactions, external energy is required for the reaction to occur and is absorbed from the surroundings. Some reactions require energy to start the reaction. This energy is called activation energy. A match applied to tissue paper is an example of activation energy. When the same number of atoms is present on the reactant side of an equation as on the product side, the reaction is said to be in equilibrium. All atoms of a substance must be accounted for after it undergoes a chemical reaction. For instance, methane reacting with oxygen produces water and carbon dioxide, but all atoms in the original substances are still present, albeit in different combinations.

Catalysis
Catalysis occurs when a catalyst is added to a reaction to increase its rate and efficiency. Catalysts change the rate of a reaction without being changed by the reaction and are important elements of chemical and biological processes. They function by decreasing the activation energy required for a reaction to occur. Homogeneous catalysis occurs when the catalyst is in the same state of matter as the reactant(s) and product(s). Heterogeneous catalysis occurs when the

catalyst is in a different state. For example, hydrogen peroxide (H_2O_2) breaks down naturally to produce water and oxygen; this is normally a very slow reaction. Liquid hydrogen bromide can be added to the H_2O_2 to speed up the reaction considerably; because all compounds in question are liquid, this is an example of homogeneous catalysis. Solid manganese dioxide crystals (MnO_2) can also be added to the H_2O_2 as a catalyst to demonstrate heterogeneous catalysis.

Types of chemical reactions

Electron transfer, or redox reactions, occurs when electrons move from one atom to another, changing the charge of the ion. Because the charge has changed, the oxidation number also changes. Oxidation is an important class of redox reactions in which the oxidation number increases. Commonly, any reaction in which oxygen combines with other substances is oxidation. Rusting iron and burning wood are both examples of oxidation.

Precipitation, or ion combination reactions, occurs when positive and negative compounds in solution combine to form an insoluble ionic compound. Acid-base reactions occur when an acid reacts with a base and an ion of hydrogen transfers to the base.

Polymerization reactions occur when simple molecules, also called monomers, combine to form complex molecules, or polymers.

Combination reactions occur when pairs of reactants combine to produce a single substance. The reactions take place when it the energy is favorable to do so. For instance:

$C(s) + O2(g) -> CO2(g)$
$N2(g) + 3H2(g) -> 2NH3(g)$
$CaO(s) + H2O(1) -> Ca(OH)2(s)$

Decomposition refers to the reaction involving those molecules which are stable at room temperature and decompose when heated:

$2KClO3(s) -> 2KCl(s) + 3O3(g)$

$PbCO3(s) -> 2PbO(s) + CO2(g)$

Single substitution is when a reaction involves an element that displaces another in a compound such as when a copper strip displaces silver atoms and produces copper nitrate and precipitating silver crystals of metal:

$Cu(s) + 2AgNO3(aq) -> 2Ag(s) + Cu(NO3)2(aq)$

Double substitution is when a reaction looks as if it is exchanging parts of the reactants. An example:

$2KI(aq) + Pb(NO3)2(aq) -> 2KNO3 (aq) + PbI(s)$

Oxidation/reduction reactions

One way to organize chemical reactions is to sort them into two categories: oxidation/reduction reactions (also called redox reactions) and metathesis reactions (which include acid/base reactions). Oxidation/reduction reactions can involve the transfer of one or more electrons, or they can occur as a result of the transfer of oxygen, hydrogen, or halogen atoms. The species that loses electrons is oxidized and is referred to as the reducing agent. The species that gains electrons is reduced and is referred to as the oxidizing agent. The element undergoing oxidation experiences an increase in its oxidation number, while the element undergoing reduction experiences a decrease in its oxidation number. Single replacement reactions are types of oxidation/reduction reactions. In a single replacement reaction, electrons are transferred from one chemical species to another. The transfer of electrons results in changes in the nature and charge of the species.

Metathesis (acid/base) reactions

Double replacement reactions are metathesis reactions. In a double replacement reaction, the chemical reactants exchange ions but the oxidation state stays the same. One of the indicators of this is the formation of a solid precipitate. In acid/base reactions, an acid is a compound that can donate a proton, while a base is a compound that can accept a proton. In these types of reactions, the acid and base react to form a salt and water. When the proton is donated, the base becomes water and the remaining ions form a salt. One method of determining whether a reaction is an oxidation/reduction or a metathesis reaction is that the oxidation number of atoms does not change during a metathesis reaction.

Oxidizing agent, reduction agent, and rate-determining step

An oxidizing agent is the reactant in oxidation reactions which gains electrons, causing oxidation of the other reactant(s). Peroxides, iodine and other halogens, and sulfoxides are common oxidizing agents. A reduction, or reducing agent, is the reactant oxidized in an oxidation reaction; it loses electrons to the oxidizing agent. In rusting iron, a common oxidation reaction, iron is the reducing agent, losing electrons to oxygen. In multi-step reactions, each of the steps has different reaction rates which are often very different. The rate-determining step is the slowest portion of such reactions. Because the reaction can only go as fast as its slowest step, that step determines overall reaction rate.

Law of Conservation of Mass

The Law of Conservation of Mass in a chemical reaction is commonly stated as follows:
In a chemical reaction, matter is neither created nor destroyed.
What this means is that there will always be the same total mass of material after a reaction as before. This allows for predicting how molecules will combine by balanced equations in which the number of each type of atom is the same on either side of the equation. For example, two hydrogen molecules combine with one oxygen molecule to form water. This is a balanced chemical equation because the number of each type of atom is same on both sides of the arrow. It has to balance because the reaction obeys the Law of Conservation of Mass.

Reading chemical equations

Chemical equations describe chemical reactions. The reactants are on the left side before the arrow and the products are on the right side after the arrow. The arrow indicates the reaction or change. The coefficient, or stoichiometric coefficient, is the number before the element, and indicates the ratio of reactants to products in terms of moles. The equation for the formation of water from hydrogen and oxygen, for example, is $2H_2$ (g) + O_2 (g) → $2H_2O$ (l). The 2 preceding hydrogen and water is the coefficient, which means there are 2 moles of hydrogen and 2 of water. There is 1 mole of oxygen, which does not have to be indicated with the number 1. In parentheses, g stands for gas, l stands for liquid, s stands for solid, and aq stands for aqueous solution (a substance dissolved in water). Charges are shown in superscript for individual ions, but not for ionic compounds. Polyatomic ions are separated by parentheses so the ion will not be confused with the number of ions.

Hydrocarbons

Hydrocarbons are molecules containing only C and H and form the basis of organic chemistry. They bond together with strong covalent bonds in chains or rings to form the backbone of organic molecules which may have any number of a large variety of functional groups attached. Hydrocarbons are classified into two large groups based on the bonds between their C atoms; if only C—C single bonds are present, the hydrocarbon is saturated because other electrons will then form bonds with surrounding H atoms. If the C atoms are bound with multiple bonds (C=C or CÐC), fewer electrons are available to form bonds

- 61 -

with H atoms and the hydrocarbon is unsaturated. Hydrocarbons are very stable molecules because of the tetravalency of C; it has four valence electrons making its octet requirement easy to satisfy, which results in very strong bonds.

Mixture, heterogeneous mixture, homogeneous mixture, and pure substance

A mixture is made of two or more substances that are combined in various proportions with each retaining its own specific properties. A mixture's components may be separated by physical means, without making and breaking chemical bonds. An example would be table salt being completely dissolved in water. Heterogeneous mixtures are those in which the composition and properties are not uniform throughout the entire sample. Examples include concrete and wood. Homogeneous mixtures are those in which the composition and properties are uniform throughout the entire sample. Pure substances are those substances with composition that is constant. They may fit the classification as either a compound or an element.

Bases

Basic chemicals are usually in aqueous solution and have the following traits: a bitter taste; a soapy or slippery texture to the touch; the capacity to restore the blue color of litmus paper which had previously been turned red by an acid; the ability to produce salts in reaction with acids.
"Alkali" is often used to describe bases. While acids yield hydrogen ions (H^+) when dissolved in solution, bases yield hydroxide ions (OH^-); the same models used to describe acids can be inverted and used to describe bases— Arrhenius, Brønsted-Lowry, and Lewis.

Some nonmetal oxides (such as Na_2O) are classified as bases even though they do not contain hydroxides in their molecular form. However, these substances easily produce hydroxide ions when reacted with water, which is why they are classified as bases.

Acids

Acids are a unique class of compounds characterized by consistent properties. The most significant property of an acid is not readily observable and is what gives acids their unique behaviors: the ionization of H atoms, or their tendency to dissociate from their parent molecules and take on an electrical charge. Carboxylic acids are also characterized by ionization, but of the O atoms. Some other properties of acids are easy to observe without any experimental apparatus. These properties include the following:

- A sour taste
- Change the color of litmus paper to red
- Produce gaseous H_2 in reaction with some metals
- Produce salt precipitates in reaction with bases

Other properties, while no more complex, are less easily observed. For instance, most inorganic acids are easily soluble in water and have high boiling points.

Strong or weak acids and bases

The characteristic properties of acids and bases derive from the tendency of atoms to ionize by donating or accepting charged particles. The strength of an acid or base is a reflection of the degree to which its atoms ionize in solution. For example, if all of the atoms in an acid ionize, the acid is said to be strong. When only a few of the atoms ionize, the acid is weak. Acetic acid ($HC_2H_3O_2$) is a weak acid because only its O2 atoms ionize in

- 62 -

solution. Another way to think of the strength of an acid or base is to consider its reactivity. Highly reactive acids and bases are strong because they tend to form and break bonds quickly and most of their atoms ionize in the process.

Dissolve, solute, solvent, solution, and solubility

To dissolve is to reduce a compound to smaller and smaller sizes until it is distributed evenly and interacts on a molecular level with the solvent in a solution. Solute is the target substance or substances dissolved in a solution; a teaspoon of sugar may be the solute in a cup of tea. Solvent is the medium in which the solute is dissolved, such as the water in saltwater. A solution is the mixture of a solvent and its solute(s). Solutions are homogeneous and symmetrical because any portion of a solution has the same composition and contents of any other portion. Components of solutions can be separated from each other but not through simple means like filtration. When the concentration of a solute is constant, the solution is saturated. Unsaturated solution simply has less solute. Solubility is the amount of a substance that dissolves in a solvent.

Enzymes

Enzymes are proteins with strong catalytic power. They greatly accelerate the speed at which specific reactions approach equilibrium. Although enzymes do not start chemical reactions that would not eventually occur by themselves, they do make these reactions happen faster and more often. This acceleration can be substantial, sometimes making reactions happen a million times faster. Each type of enzyme deals with reactants, also called substrates. Each enzyme is highly selective, only interacting with substrates that are a match for it at an active site on the enzyme. This is the "key in the lock"

analogy: a certain enzyme only fits with certain substrates. Because of this selectivity, the fit is not always perfect. An unusual quality of enzymes is that they are not permanently consumed in the reactions they speed up. They can be used again and again, providing a constant source of energy accelerants for cells. This allows for a tremendous increase in the number and rate of reactions in cells.

Energy

Some discussions of energy consider only two types of energy: kinetic energy (the energy of motion) and potential energy (which depends on relative position). There are, however, other types of energy. Electromagnetic waves, for example, are a type of energy contained by a field. Gravitational energy is a form of potential energy. Objects perched any distance from the ground have gravitational energy, or the potential to move. Another type of potential energy is electrical energy, which is the energy it takes to pull apart positive and negative electrical charges. Chemical energy refers to the manner in which atoms form into molecules, and this energy can be released or absorbed when molecules regroup. Solar energy comes in the form of visible light and non-visible light, such as infrared and ultraviolet rays. Sound energy refers to the energy in sound waves.

Kinetic and potential energy
Kinetic and potential energy are two commonly known types of energy. Kinetic energy refers to the energy of an object in motion. The following formula is used to calculate kinetic energy: $KE = \frac{1}{2} mv^2$, where "KE" stands for kinetic energy, "m" stands for mass, and "v" stands for velocity. Even though an object may appear to be motionless, its atoms are always moving. Since these atoms are colliding and moving, they have kinetic

energy. Potential energy refers to a capacity for doing work that is based upon position or configuration. The following formula can be used to calculate potential energy: PE = mgh, where "PE" stands for potential energy, "m" stands for mass, "g" stands for gravity, and "h" stands for height.

Chemical potential energy and electromagnetic potential energy

Everything has molecules. Energy is required to make these molecules and hold them together. The energy stored in molecules is called chemical potential energy. An example is the energy stored in gasoline. Bonds are broken and reformed during combustion and new products are made. The energy stored in gasoline is released when it is burned, which is combustion. Gasoline is changed into byproducts during combustion such as water and carbon dioxide, and energy is released. An airplane motor will use the energy that is released to turn a propeller. A battery has chemical potential energy as well as electrical potential energy. When a flashlight is turned on, the electrical potential energy stored in the battery is converted into other forms of energy such as light. With an electrical appliance that is plugged in, electrical potential energy is maintained in a power plant's generator, a windmill or a hydroelectric dam.

Properties of water

The important properties of water (H_2O) are high polarity, hydrogen bonding, cohesiveness, adhesiveness, high specific heat, high latent heat, and high heat of vaporization. It is essential to life as we know it, as water is one of the main if not the main constituent of many living things. Water is a liquid at room temperature. The high specific heat of water means it resists the breaking of its hydrogen bonds and resists heat and motion, which is why it has a relatively high boiling point and high vaporization point. It also resists temperature change. In its solid state, water floats. Most substances are heavier in their solid forms. Water is cohesive, which means it is attracted to itself. It is also adhesive, which means it readily attracts other molecules. If water tends to adhere to another substance, the substance is said to be hydrophilic. Water makes a good solvent. Substances, particularly those with polar ions and molecules, readily dissolve in water.

Catalysts and the Maxwell-Boltzmann distribution

Catalysts, substances that help change the rate of reaction without changing their form, can increase reaction rate by decreasing the number of steps it takes to form products. The mass of the catalyst should be the same at the beginning of the reaction as it is at the end. The activation energy is the minimum amount required to get a reaction started. Activation energy causes particles to collide with sufficient energy to start the reaction. A catalyst enables more particles to react, which lowers the activation energy. Examples of catalysts in reactions are manganese oxide (MnO_2) in the decomposition of hydrogen peroxide, iron in the manufacture of ammonia using the Haber process, and concentrate of sulfuric acid in the nitration of benzene. Maxwell-Boltzmann distribution: This refers to a graph or plot showing the energies or speeds of particles or gas molecules in a system.

PH

The potential of hydrogen (pH) is a measurement of the concentration of hydrogen ions in a substance in terms of the number of moles of H^+ per liter of solution. All substances fall between 0 and 14 on the pH scale. A lower pH indicates a higher H^+ concentration, while

- 64 -

a higher pH indicates a lower H⁺ concentration. Pure water has a neutral pH, which is 7. Anything with a pH lower than water (0 to 6) is considered acidic. Anything with a pH higher than water (8 to 14) is a base. Drain cleaner, soap, baking soda, ammonia, egg whites, and sea water are common bases. Urine, stomach acid, citric acid, vinegar, hydrochloric acid, and battery acid are acids. A pH indicator is a substance that acts as a detector of hydrogen or hydronium ions. It is halochromic, meaning it changes color to indicate that hydrogen or hydronium ions have been detected.

Sun

Features and characteristics
The Sun is at the center of the solar system. It is composed of 70% hydrogen (H) and 28% helium (He). The remaining 2% is made up of metals. The Sun is one of 100 billion stars in the Milky Way galaxy. Its diameter is 1,390,000 km, its mass is 1.989×10^{30} kg, its surface temperature is 5,800 K, and its core temperature is 15,600,000 K. The Sun represents more than 99.8% of the total mass of the solar system. At the core, the temperature is 15.6 million K, the pressure is 250 billion atmospheres, and the density is more than 150 times that of water. The surface is called the photosphere. The chromosphere lies above this, and the corona, which extends millions of kilometers into space, is next. Sunspots are relatively cool regions on the surface with a temperature of 3,800 K. Temperatures in the corona are over 1,000,000 K. Its magnetosphere, or heliosphere, extends far beyond Pluto.

Energy
The Sun's energy is produced by nuclear fusion reactions. Each second, about 700,000,000 tons of hydrogen are converted (or fused) to about 695,000,000 tons of helium and

5,000,000 tons of energy in the form of gamma rays. In nuclear fusion, four hydrogen nuclei are fused into one helium nucleus, resulting in the release of energy. In the Sun, the energy proceeds towards the surface and is absorbed and re-emitted at lower and lower temperatures. Energy is mostly in the form of visible light when it reaches the surface. It is estimated that the Sun has used up about half of the hydrogen at its core since its birth. It is expected to radiate in this fashion for another 5 billion years. Eventually, it will deplete its hydrogen fuel, grow brighter, expand to about 260 times its diameter, and become a red giant. The outer layers will ablate and become a dense white dwarf the size of the Earth.

Renewable energy: Renewable energy can be used without being used up. Most of it comes from the Sun and its effects on Earth. Examples:
- Solar power - Active and passive solar heating of water and building materials uses the Sun's energy directly. Solar energy also can be captured and concentrated to make steam to run electricity-generating turbines or for use in solar cookers. Photovoltaic (solar) cells can convert sunlight to electricity.
- Biomass - The Sun's energy is stored in trees and other plants and in plant and animal wastes that we can burn or process to make biofuels, such as biodiesel.
- Hydropower - The water cycle is powered by the Sun. The kinetic energy in water moving through the cycle can be converted to electricity with dams and by small-scale hydroelectric machinery in flowing rivers. There are also devices to harvest the movement of tides and waves.

Important terms

- Atom - An atom is one of the most basic units of matter. An atom consists of a central nucleus surrounded by electrons.
- Nucleus - The nucleus of an atom consists of protons and neutrons. It is positively charged, dense, and heavier than the surrounding electrons. The plural form of nucleus is nuclei.
- Electrons - These are atomic particles that are negatively charged and orbit the nucleus of an atom.
- Protons - Along with neutrons, protons make up the nucleus of an atom. The number of protons in the nucleus usually determines the atomic number of an element. Carbon atoms, for example, have six protons. The atomic number of carbon is 6. The number of protons also indicates the charge of an atom.
- Atomic number (proton number) - The atomic number of an element, also known as the proton number, refers to the number of protons in the nucleus of an atom. It is a unique identifier. It can be represented as "Z." Atoms with a neutral charge have an atomic number that is equal to the number of electrons. The number of protons in the atomic nucleus also determines its electric charge, which in turn determines the number of electrons the atom has in its non-ionized state.
- Neutrons - Neutrons are the uncharged atomic particles contained within the nucleus. The number of neutrons in a nucleus can be represented as "N."
- Nucleon - This refers to the collective number of neutrons and protons.

- Element - An element is matter with one type of atom. It can be identified by its atomic number. There are 117 elements, 94 of which occur naturally on Earth.

Scientific Reasoning

Scientific method of inquiry

The scientific method of inquiry is a general method by which ideas are tested and either confirmed or refuted by experimentation. The first step in the scientific method is formulating the problem that is to be addressed. It is essential to clearly define the limits of what is to be observed, since that allows for a more focused analysis. Once the problem has been defined, it is necessary to form a hypothesis. This educated guess should be a possible solution to the problem that was formulated in the first step. The next step is to test that hypothesis by experimentation. This often requires the scientist to design a complete experiment. The key to making the best possible use of an experiment is observation. Observations may be quantitative, that is, when a numeric measurement is taken, or they may be qualitative, that is, when something is evaluated based on feeling or preference. This measurement data will then be examined to find trends or patterns that are present. From these trends, the scientist will then draw conclusions or make generalizations about the results, intended to predict future results. If these conclusions support the original hypothesis, the experiment is complete and the scientist will publish his conclusions to allow others to test them by repeating the experiment. If they do not support the hypothesis, the results should then be used to develop a new hypothesis, which can then be verified by a new or redesigned experiment.

Scientific process skills

Perhaps the most important skill in science is that of observation. A scientist must be able to take accurate data from his experimental setup or from nature without allowing bias to alter the results. Another important skill is hypothesizing. A scientist must be able to combine his knowledge of theory and of other experimental results to logically determine what should occur in his own tests. The data-analysis process requires the twin skills of ordering and categorizing. Gathered data must be arranged in such a way that it is readable and readily shows the key results. A skill that may be integrated with the previous two is comparing. A scientist should be able to compare his own results with other published results. He must also be able to infer, or draw logical conclusions, from his results. He must be able to apply his knowledge of theory and results to create logical experimental designs and determine cases of special behavior. Lastly, a scientist must be able to communicate his results and his conclusions. The greatest scientific progress is made when scientists are able to review and test one another's work and offer advice or suggestions.

Scientific statements

Hypotheses are educated guesses about what is likely to occur, and are made to provide a starting point from which to begin design of the experiment. They may be based on results of previously observed experiments or knowledge of theory, and follow logically forth from these. Assumptions are statements that are taken to be fact without proof for the purpose of performing a given experiment. They may be entirely true, or they may be true only for a given set of conditions under which the experiment will be conducted. Assumptions are necessary to simplify experiments;

indeed, many experiments would be impossible without them. Scientific models are mathematical statements that describe a physical behavior. Models are only as good as our knowledge of the actual system. Often models will be discarded when new discoveries are made that show the model to be inaccurate. While a model can never perfectly represent an actual system, they are useful for simplifying a system to allow for better understanding of its behavior. Scientific laws are statements of natural behavior that have stood the test of time and have been found to produce accurate and repeatable results in all testing. A theory is a statement of behavior that consolidates all current observations. Theories are similar to laws in that they describe natural behavior, but are more recently developed and are more susceptible to being proved wrong. Theories may eventually become laws if they stand up to scrutiny and testing.

Experimental design

Designing relevant experiments that allow for meaningful results is not a simple task. Every stage of the experiment must be carefully planned to ensure that the right data can be safely and accurately taken. Ideally, an experiment should be controlled so that all of the conditions except the ones being manipulated are held constant. This helps to ensure that the results are not skewed by unintended consequences of shifting conditions. A good example of this is a placebo group in a drug trial. All other conditions are the same, but that group is not given the medication. In addition to proper control, it is important that the experiment be designed with data collection in mind. For instance, if the quantity to be measured is temperature, there must be a temperature device such as a thermocouple integrated into the experimental setup. While the data are being collected, they should periodically be checked for obvious errors. If there are data points that are orders of magnitude from the expected value, then it might be a good idea to make sure that no experimental errors are being made, either in data collection or condition control. Once all the data have been gathered, they must be analyzed. The way in which this should be done depends on the type of data and the type of trends observed. It may be useful to fit curves to the data to determine if the trends follow a common mathematical form. It may also be necessary to perform a statistical analysis of the results to determine what effects are significant. Data should be clearly presented.

Changing nature of scientific knowledge

Perhaps the greatest peculiarity of scientific knowledge is that, at the same time that it is taken as fact, it may be disproved. Current scientific knowledge is the basis from which new discoveries are made. Yet even knowledge that has stood for hundreds of years is not considered too infallible to be challenged. If someone can create an experiment whose results consistently and reproducibly defy a law that has been in place for generations, that law will be nullified. It is absolutely essential, however, that these reproductions of the experiment be conducted by many different scientists who are in isolation from one another so there is no bias or interacting effects on the results.

Applications of science and technology

Scientific and technological developments have led to the widespread availability of technologies heretofore unheard of, including cellular phones, satellite-based applications, and a worldwide network of connected computers. Some of the notable recent applications include:

- Health care: Antibiotics, genetic screening for diseases, the sequencing of the human genome. Issues include problems with health care distribution on an increasingly industrialized planet.
- The environment: Computerized models of climate change and pollution monitoring. Issues include increased pollution of the water, air, and soil, and the over-harvesting of natural resources with mechanized equipment.
- Agriculture: Genetic improvements in agricultural practices, including increased output on the same amount of arable land. Issues include unknown environmental effects of hybrid species, cross-pollination with organic species, and pollution caused by synthetic chemical fertilizers.
- Information technology: New Internet-based industries, increased worldwide collaboration, and access to information. Issues include the depletion of natural resources for electronics production.

Social impacts of recent developments in science and technology

Recent developments in science and technology have had both positive and negative effects on human society. The issue of sustainable growth is an increasingly important one, as humans realize that the resources they use are not unlimited. Genetic research into diseases, stem cell research, and cloning technology have created great controversies as they have been introduced, and an increasing number of people reject the morality of scientific practices like animal testing in the pursuit of scientific advancement. In addition, an increasingly technology-based world has produced a new social inequality based on access to computers and Internet technology.

These issues are beginning to be debated at all levels of human government, from city councils to the United Nations. Does science provide the authoritative answer to all human problems, or do ethics carry weight in scientific debates as well? Ultimately, humans must weigh the competing needs of facilitating scientific pursuits and maintaining an ethical society as they face new technological questions.

English and Language Usage

Grammar and Word Meanings in Context

Grammar

Grammar may be practically defined as the study of how words are put together or the study of sentences. There are multiple approaches to grammar in modern linguistics. Any systematic account of the structure of a language and the patterns it describes is grammar. Modern definitions state that grammar is the knowledge of a language developed in the minds of the speakers.

A grammar, in the broadest sense, is a set of rules internalized by members of a speech community, and an account, by a linguist, of such a grammar. This internalized grammar is what is commonly called a language. Grammar is often restricted to units that have meaning. The expanded scope of grammar includes morphology and syntax and a lexicon. Grammatical meaning is described as part of the syntax and morphology of a language, as distinct from its lexicon.

Words and tone

A writer's choice of words is a signature of his or her style. A careful analysis of the use of words can improve a piece of writing. Attention to the use of specific nouns rather than general ones can enliven language. Verbs should be active whenever possible to keep the writing stronger and energetic, and there should be an appropriate balance between numbers of nouns and verbs. Too many nouns can result in heavy, boring sentences.

Tone may be defined as the writer's attitude toward the topic, and to the audience. This attitude is reflected in the language used in the writing. The tone of a work should be appropriate to the topic and to the intended audience. Some writing should avoid slang and jargon although it may be fine in a different piece. Tone can range from humorous to serious and all levels in between. It may be more or less formal, depending on the purpose of the writing and its intended audience. All these nuances in tone can flavor the entire writing and should be kept in mind as the work evolves.

Phonology

General phonetics classifies the speech sounds of all languages. Any one language uses only some of the possibilities of the selections available. Sounds and how they are used in a language is the phonology of a language. Dynamic features of phonology include speech melody, stress, rhythmic organization, length, and syllabicity. The central unit of phonology is the phoneme, the smallest distinct sound in a given language.

Two words are composed of different phonemes only if they differ phonetically in ways that are found to make a difference in meaning. Phonemic transcription of a word or phrase is its representation as a sequence or other combinations of phonemes.

Phonology is a controversial and enigmatic part of linguistics. It is widely studied and defined, but there is no agreement on the definition of a phoneme or phonology theory. There may be as many theories as there are phonologies in linguistics.

Morphology

Morphology is the grammatical structure of words and their categories. The morphological process includes any of the formal processes or operations by which the forms of words are derived from stems or roots. Types of morphological processes include affix, any element in the structure of a word other than a root; reduplication, where all or part of a form is duplicated; subtraction, where part of a form is deleted; suppletion, where one part of the morphological process replaces another; compound, where two parts of the morphological process are joined; and modification, where one part of a form is modified.

Forms of morphological classification:

- distinguished isolating - each grammatical classification is represented by a single word
- agglutinating - words are easily divided into separate
- sections inflectional - concerned with inflections in languages

Etymology

Etymology is the study of the historical relation between a word and earlier form or forms from which it has developed. Etymology can be loosely defined as the study of the origins of words. This study may occur on different levels of linguistic approach. Word meanings and their historical antecedents are often a complicated and controversial source of study. Tracing the meaning of words often includes understanding the social, political, and cultural time that the definition existed. The evolution of words from earlier forms suggests a cross-fertilization of social contexts and common usage that is a fascinating field of study.

An etymological fallacy is that the notion that a true meaning of a word can be derived from its etymology. Modern linguistic theory provides a substantial body of knowledge that compares and evaluates etymology and provides numerous avenues for new research.

Nouns and pronouns

Nouns name persons, places, things, animals, objects, time, feelings, concepts, and actions, and are usually signaled by an article (a, an, the). Nouns sometimes function as adjectives modifying other nouns. Nouns used in this manner are called noun/adjectives. Nouns are classified for a number of purposes: capitalization, word choice, count/no count nouns, and collective nouns are examples.

A pronoun is a word used in place of a noun. Usually the pronoun substitutes for the specific noun, called the antecedent. Although most pronouns function as substitutes for nouns, some can function as adjectives modifying nouns. Pronouns may be classed as personal, possessive, intensive, relative (*which, that, who, whoever*), interrogative, demonstrative (*this, that, these, those*), indefinite (*anybody, somebody, everybody*), and reciprocal. Personal pronouns (*he, she, they*) refer to specific people, places, or things and can be either singular or plural. Possessive pronouns (*his, hers, theirs, ours*) are used to show ownership. Pronouns can cause a number of problems for writers, including pronoun-antecedent agreement, distinguishing between who and whom, and differentiating pronouns, such as I and me.

Functions of pronouns

A *pronoun* always refers back to a noun. That noun is the pronoun's antecedent. Example: She bought some (antecedent) furniture yesterday, but (pronoun) it hasn't arrived. Pronoun and antecedent must agree in number and gender. Example: We were happy when our (antecedent) relatives came. It was great seeing (pronoun) them.

A *personal pronoun* refers to a person or thing. A personal pronoun can be a subject, an object, or a possessive. Personal pronouns usually change their form depending on if they are used as the subject or object of a sentence.

1st Person: I, we, me, us, mine, ours
2nd Person: you, yours
3rd Person: he, she, it, they, him, her, them, his, hers, theirs

Interrogative pronouns (who, whom, which, what, and whose) ask questions. *Relative pronouns* (who, whom, which, that, whose) introduce adjective and noun clauses. The relative pronoun, what, introduces noun clauses only. Within an adjective or noun clause, the relative pronoun can function as a subject, object, or possessive. Relative pronouns of the -ever form (whatever, whichever, whoever, whomever) have an indefinite meaning: they do not refer back to a specific noun.

Problems with pronouns
Pronouns are words that substitute for nouns: he, it, them, her, me, and so on. Four frequently encountered problems with pronouns include the following:

- Pronoun-antecedent agreement: The antecedent of a pronoun is the word the pronoun refers to. A pronoun and its antecedent agree when they are both singular or plural, or of the same gender.
- Pronoun reference: A pronoun should refer clearly to its antecedent. A pronoun's reference will be unclear if it is ambiguous, implied, vague, or indefinite.
- Personal pronouns: Some pronouns change their case form according to their grammatical structure in a sentence. Pronouns functioning as subjects appear in the subjective case, those functioning as objects appear in the objective case, and those functioning as possessives appear in the possessive case.
- Who or whom: *Who*, a subjective-case pronoun, can be used only as subjects and subject

complements. *Whom*, an objective-case pronoun, can be used only for objects. The words *who* and *whom* appear primarily in subordinate clauses or in questions.

Pronoun-antecedent agreement
An antecedent is the word or phrase to which a pronoun refers. An antecedent must come before a pronoun in a sentence, and a pronoun and its antecedent must agree. Plural antecedents require plural pronouns, while singular antecedents require singular pronouns. The antecedent and pronoun must also agree in gender and person, as in the following examples: The <u>man</u> used <u>his</u> glasses. The <u>three children</u> were eating <u>their</u> ice cream. In the first example, *man* is the antecedent, and *his* is the pronoun. In the second example, *three children* is the antecedent, while *their* is the pronoun. In both examples, antecedents and pronouns agree in gender and person.

Noun-pronoun agreement in number
A pronoun must agree with its antecedent in number. If the antecedent is singular, the pronoun referring to it must be singular; if the antecedent is plural, the pronoun referring to it must be plural.
- Use singular pronouns to refer to the singular indefinite pronouns: *each, either, neither, one, everyone, everybody, no one, nobody, anyone, anybody, someone, somebody.*
Example: Each of the students bought their own lunch. (incorrect)
            Each of the students bought his own lunch. (correct)
- Use plural nouns to refer to the plural indefinite pronouns: *both, few, several, many.*
Example: *Both* were within *their* boundaries.
- The indefinite pronouns *some, any, none, all, most* may be referred to by singular or

plural pronouns, depending on the sense of the sentence.

Examples: *Some* of the children have misplaced *their* toy. (plural)

Some of the carpet has lost *its* nap. (singular)

- Pronouns that refer to compound antecedents joined by and are usually plural.

Example: Bill and Joe cook *their* own meals.

Pronoun-noun agreement in gender

A pronoun agrees with its antecedent in gender.

- Antecedents of *masculine* gender (male sex) are referred to by *he, him, his*.
- Antecedents of *feminine* gender (female sex) are referred to by *she, her, hers*.
- Antecedents of *neuter* gender (no sex) are referred to by *it, its*.
- Antecedents of *common* gender (sex not known) are referred to by *he, him, his*. It is understood that the masculine pronouns include both male and female.
- Antecedents that are names of animals are generally referred to by the neuter pronouns unless the writer wishes to indicate special interest in the animal, in which case the masculine pronouns are often used. When a feminine role is naturally suggested, the feminine pronouns are used.

Adjectives, articles, and adverbs

An adjective is a word used to modify or describe a noun or pronoun. An adjective usually answers one of these questions: Which one? What kind? How many? Adjectives usually precede the words they modify although they sometimes follow linking verbs, in which case they describe the subject.

Articles, sometimes classed as nouns, are used to mark nouns. There are only three: the definite article the and the indefinite articles a and an.

An adverb is a word used to modify or qualify a verb, adjective, or another adverb. It usually answers one of these questions: When? Where? How? Why? Adverbs modifying adjectives or other adverbs usually intensify or limit the intensity of words they modify. The negators not and never are classified as adverbs.

Writers sometimes misuse adverbs, and multilingual speakers have trouble placing them correctly.

Verbs

The verb of a sentence usually expresses action or being. It is composed of a main verb and sometimes supporting verbs. These helping verbs are forms of have, do, and be, and nine modals. The modals are can, could, may, might, shall, should, will, would, and ought. Some verbs are followed by words that look like prepositions but are so closely associated with the verb as to be part of its meaning. These words are known as particles, and examples include call off, look up, and drop off.

The main verb of a sentence is always one that would change form from base form to past tense, past participle, present participle, and –s forms. When both the past-tense and past-participle forms of a verb end in –ed, the verb is regular. In all other cases, the verb is irregular. The verb to be is highly irregular, having eight forms instead of the usual five.

Prepositions and conjunctions

A preposition is a word placed before a noun or pronoun to form a phrase modifying another word in the sentence. The prepositional phrase usually functions as an adjective or adverb. There are a limited number of prepositions in English, perhaps around 80. Some prepositions are more than one word long. Along with, listen to, and next to are some examples.

Conjunctions join words, phrases, or clauses, and they indicate the relationship between the elements that are joined. There are coordinating conjunctions that connect grammatically equal elements, correlative conjunctions that connect pairs, subordinating conjunctions that introduce a subordinate clause, and conjunctive adverbs, which may be used with a semicolon to connect independent clauses. The most common conjunctive adverbs include then, thus, and however. Using conjunctions correctly helps avoid sentence fragments and run-on sentences.

Subject-verb agreement

In the present tense, verbs agree with their subjects in number, (singular or plural) and in person (first, second, or third). The present tense ending –s is used with a verb if its subject is third person singular; otherwise, the verb takes no ending. The verb to be varies from this pattern, and, alone among verbs, it has special forms in both the present and past tense.

Problems with subject-verb agreement tend to arise in certain contexts:

- Words between subject and verbs
- Subjects joined by and
- Subjects joined by or or nor
- Indefinite pronouns, such as someone
- Collective nouns
- Subject after the verb
- Pronouns who, which, and that
- Plural form, singular meaning
- Titles, company names, and words mentioned as words

Common grammatical mistakes
Subjects and verbs must agree in number. Often students, particularly those rushing to complete a test, make errors in subject-verb agreement. Even if the subject and verb of a sentence are separated by other words, they should still agree in number. Singular subjects require singular verbs, while plural subjects require plural verbs. Sometimes a subject will be a collective noun that represents a group. If the group acts as a single being, a singular verb should be used. If the group acts separately, a plural verb should be used. When there are two subjects separated by the word and, a plural verb should be used. When multiple subjects are separated by or, either/or, or neither/nor, a singular verb should be used.

Indefinite pronouns
The rules of subject-verb agreement state that singular subjects need singular verb forms, while plural subjects need plural verb forms. This rule seems simple, but it can become confusing when sentences have complex structures. For indefinite pronouns (whoever, anyone, someone, everyone, everybody), the writer should use singular verb forms. For the indefinite pronouns all and some, whether the writer should use a singular or plural verb form depends on what the pronoun is referring to. The indefinite pronoun none can be used with either a singular or plural verb form. In this case, another word in the sentence may help the writer determine which form to use. For example, in the sentence "None of the towels are clean," the indefinite pronoun none refers to towels, so the verb takes a plural form. In the sentence "None of the building is repaired," none refers to the building, which is singular, and so the verb becomes singular.

Subject of a sentence

The subject of a sentence names who or what the sentence is about. The complete subject is composed of the simple subject and all of its modifiers.

To find the complete subject, ask who or what. Insert the verb to complete the question. The answer is the complete subject. To find the simple subject, strip away all the modifiers in the complete subject.

In imperative sentences, the verb's subject is understood, but not actually present in the sentence. Although the subject ordinarily comes before the verb, in sentences that begin with *There are* or *There was*, the subject follows the verb. The ability to recognize the subject of a sentence helps in editing a variety of problems, such as sentence fragments and subject-verb agreement, as well as the choice of pronouns.

Drama

Dramatic dialogue

Dramatic dialogue can be difficult to interpret and changes depending upon the tone used and which words are emphasized. Where the stresses, or meters, of dramatic dialogue fall can determine meaning. Variations in emphasis are only one factor in the manipulability of dramatic speech. Tone is of equal or greater importance and expresses a range of possible emotions and feelings that cannot be readily discerned from the script of a play. The reader must add tone to the words to understand the full meaning of a passage. Recognizing tone is a cumulative process as the reader begins to understand the characters and situations in the play. Other elements that influence the interpretation of dialogue include the setting, possible reactions of the characters to the speech, and possible gestures or facial expressions of the actor. There are no firm rules to guide the interpretation of dramatic speech. An open and flexible attitude is essential in interpreting dramatic dialogue.

Speech and dialogue, asides, and soliloquies

Analysis of speech and dialogue is important in the critical study of drama. Some playwrights use speech to develop their characters. Speeches may be long or

short, and written in as normal prose or blank verse. Some characters have a unique way of speaking which illuminates aspects of the drama. Emphasis and tone are both important, as well. Does the author make clear the tone in which lines are to be spoken, or is this open to interpretation? Sometimes there are various possibilities in tone with regard to delivering lines.

Asides and soliloquies can be important in plot and character development. Asides indicate that not all characters are privy to the lines. This may be a method of advancing or explaining the plot in a subtle manner. Soliloquies are opportunities for character development, plot enhancement, and to give insight to characters motives, feelings, and emotions. Careful study of these elements provides a reader with an abundance of clues to the major themes and plot of the work.

Prose fiction

Many elements influence a work of prose fiction. Some important ones are:

- Speech and dialogue: Characters may speak for themselves or through the narrator. Dialogue may be realistic or fantastic, depending on the author's aim.
- Thoughts and mental processes: There may be internal dialogue used as a device for plot development or character understanding.
- Dramatic involvement: Some narrators encourage readers to become involved in the events of the story, whereas others attempt to distance readers through literary devices.
- Action: This is any information that advances the plot or involves new interactions between the characters.

- Duration: The time frame of the work may be long or short, and the relationship between described time and narrative time may vary.
- Setting and description: Is the setting critical to the plot or characters? How are the action scenes described?
- Themes: This is any point of view or topic given sustained attention.
- Symbolism: Authors often veil meanings through imagery and other literary constructions.

Point of view

Point of view is the perspective from which writing occurs. There are several possibilities:
- First person is written so that the I of the story is a participant or observer.
- Second person is a device to draw the reader in more closely. It is really a variation or refinement of the first-person narrative.
- Third person, the most traditional form of point of view, is the omniscient narrator, in which the narrative voice, presumed to be the writer's, is presumed to know everything about the characters, plot, and action. Most novels use this point of view.
- A multiple point of view is narration delivered from the perspective of several characters.

In modern writing, the stream-of-consciousness technique is often used. Developed fully by James Joyce, this technique uses an interior monologue that provides the narration through the thoughts, impressions, and fantasies of the narrator.

Context

Learning new words is important to and part of comprehending and integrating unfamiliar information. When a reader encounters a new word, he can stop and find it in the dictionary or the glossary of terms but sometimes those reference tools aren't readily available or using them at the moment is impractical (e.g., during a test). Furthermore, most readers are usually not willing to take the time. Another way to determine the meaning of a word is by considering the context in which it is being used. These indirect learning hints are called context clues. They include definitions, descriptions, examples, and restatements. Because most words are learned by listening to conversations, people use this tool all the time even if they do it unconsciously. But to be effective when reading, context clues must be used judiciously because the unfamiliar word may have several subtle variations, and therefore the context clues could be misinterpreted.

Context refers to how a word is used in a sentence. Identifying context can help determine the definition of unknown words. There are different contextual clues such as definition, description, example, comparison, and contrast. The following are examples:
- Definition: the unknown word is clearly defined by the previous words. - "When he was painting, his instrument was a ___." (paintbrush)
- Description: the unknown word is described by the pervious words. - "I was hot, tired, and thirsty; I was ___." (dehydrated)
- Example: the unknown word is part of a series of examples. - "Water, soda, and ___ were the offered beverages." (coffee)
- Comparison: the unknown word is compared to another word. -

"Barney is agreeable and happy like his __ parents." (positive)

- Contrast: the unknown word is contrasted with another word. - "I prefer cold weather to __ conditions." (hot)

On standardized tests, as well as in everyday life, students are faced with words with which they are not familiar. In most cases, the definition of an unknown word can be derived from context clues. The term "context clues" refers to the ways or manner in which a word is used. When reading a passage, students should carefully examine the unfamiliar word and the words and sentences that surround it. The writer may have provided a definition in parentheses following the word, or the writer may have provided a synonym. Synonyms are useful because they offer a common substitute for the unfamiliar word. Also, the author may have provided an antonym, or opposite, for the unfamiliar word. Finally, a context clue might be found in the prior or later restatement of the idea that contained the word, and sometimes the writer may have even provided a detailed explanation of the unfamiliar word.

Synonyms, antonyms, and homonyms

Synonyms are two different words that mean the same thing. They can often be substituted for each other in sentences. For example, "pretty" is a synonym for "beautiful." Antonyms are words that have opposite meanings. For example, "ugly" is an antonym for "beautiful." Homonyms are words that are spelled or pronounced the same but have different meanings. For example, "lead" (pronounced "led") is a noun that describes a type of element. "Lead," also pronounced "led," is also the past tense form of the verb "lead," pronounced

"leed." Most homonyms are spelled differently, such as "to" and "too."

Appositive

An appositive is a word or phrase that restates or modifies an immediately preceding noun. An appositive is often useful as a context clue for determining or refining the meaning of the word or words to which it refers. For example, "My dad, whose name is James Brown, (appositive) is a lawyer."

Word usage

Word usage, or diction, refers to the use of words with meanings and forms that are appropriate for the context and structure of a sentence. A common error in word usage occurs when a word's meaning does not fit the context of the sentence.
Incorrect: Susie likes chips better then candy.
Correct: Susie likes chips better than candy.
Incorrect: The cat licked it's colt.
Correct: the cat licked its colt.
Commonly misused words include *than/then, it's/its, they/their/they're, your/you're, except/accept, and affect/effect.*

Prefixes

ab : from, away, off : abdicate, abjure
ad : to, toward : advance
ante : before, previous : antecedent, antedate
anti : against, opposing : antipathy, antidote
de : from : depart
epi : upon : epilogue
hyper : excessive, over : hypercritical, hypertension
hypo : under, beneath : hypodermic, hypothesis
inter : among, between : intercede, interrupt

intra : within : intramural, intrastate
mal : bad, poorly, not : malfunction
mor : die, death : mortality, mortuary
ob : against, opposing : objection
omni : all, everywhere : omniscient
pan : all, entire : panorama, pandemonium
per : through : perceive, permit
pre : before, previous : prevent, preclude
pro : forward, in place of : propel, pronoun
super : above, extra : supersede, supernumerary
supra : above, over: supraorbital, suprasegmental
trans : across, beyond, over : transact, transport
uni : one : uniform, unity

Suffixes

Sometimes adding a suffix can change the spelling of a root word. If the suffix begins with a vowel, the final consonant of the root word must be doubled. This rule applies only if the root word has one syllable or if the accent is on the last syllable.
For example, when adding the suffix -*ery* to the root word *rob*, the final word becomes *robbery*. The letter *b* is doubled because *rob* has only one syllable. However, when adding the suffix -*able* to the root word *profit*, the final word becomes *profitable*. The letter i is not doubled because the root word *profit* has two syllables.
Spelling is not changed when the suffixes -*less, -ness, -ly*, or -*en* are used. The only exception to this rule occurs when the suffix -*ness* or -*ly* is added to a root word ending in *y*. In this case, the *y* changes to *i*. For example, *happy* becomes *happily*.
Suffixes are a group of letters, placed behind a root word, that carry a specific meaning. Suffixes can perform one of two possible functions. They can be used to create a new word, or they can shift the tense of a word without changing its original meaning.

For example, the suffix -*ability* can be added to the end of the word *account* to form the new word *accountability*. *Account* means a written narrative or description of events, while *accountability* means the state of being liable. The suffix -*ed* can be added to *account* to form the word *accounted*, which simply shifts the word from present tense to past tense.

Certain suffixes require that the root word be modified. If the suffix begins with a vowel, such as -ing, and the root word ends in the letter e, the letter e must be dropped before adding the suffix. For example, the word write becomes writing. If the suffix begins with a consonant instead of a vowel, the letter e at the end of the root word does not need to be dropped. For example, hope becomes hopeless. The only exceptions to this rule are the words judgment, acknowledgment, and argument. If a root word ends in the letter y and is preceded by a consonant, the y is changed to i before adding the suffix. This is true for all suffixes except those that begin with i. For example, plenty becomes plentiful.

age : process, state, rank : passage, bondage
ance : act, condition, fact : acceptance, vigilance
ard : one that does excessively : drunkard, wizard
ate : having, showing : separate, desolate
ation : action, state, result : occupation, starvation
cy : state, condition : accuracy, captaincy
en : cause to be, become : deepen, strengthen
er : one who does : teacher
ess : feminine : waitress, lioness
fic : making, causing : terrific, beatific
fy : make, cause, cause to have : glorify, fortify
ion : action, result, state : union, fusion
ist : doer, believer : monopolist, socialist
ition : action, state, result : sedition, expedition

ity : state, quality, condition : acidity, civility
ize : make, cause to be, treat with : sterilize, mechanize
logue : type of speaking or writing : prologue
ly : like, of the nature of : friendly, positively
or : doer, office, action : juror, elevator, honor
ous : marked by, given to : religious, riotous
ty : quality, state : enmity, activity
ward : in the direction of : backward, homeward

Spelling and Punctuation

Spelling rules

<u>Words ending with a consonant</u>
Usually the final consonant is doubled on a word before adding a suffix. This is the rule for single syllable words, words ending with one consonant, and multi-syllable words with the last syllable accented. For example:
- beg becomes begging (single syllable)
- shop becomes shopped (single syllable)
- add becomes adding (already ends in double consonant, do not add another "d")
- deter becomes deterring (multi-syllable, accent on last syllable)
- regret becomes regrettable (multi-syllable, accent on last syllable)
- compost becomes composting (do not add another "t" because the accent is on the first syllable)

<u>Words ending in "y" and "c"</u>
The general rule for words ending in "y" is to keep the "y" when adding a suffix if the "y" is preceded by a vowel. If the word ends in a consonant and "y," the "y" is changed to an "i" before the suffix is

added (unless the suffix itself begins with "i"). The following are examples:
- pay becomes paying (keep the "y")
- bully becomes bullied (change to "i")
- bully becomes bullying (keep the "y" because the suffix is "–ing")

If a word ends with "c" and the suffix begins with an "e," "i," or "y," the letter "k" is usually added to the end of the word. The following are examples:
- panic becomes panicky
- mimic becomes mimicking

<u>Words ending in "ie," "ei," and "e"</u>
Most words are spelled with an "i" before "e," except when they follow the letter "c" OR sound like "a." For example, the following words are spelled correctly according to these rules:
- piece, friend, believe ("i" before "e")
- receive, ceiling, conceited (except after "c")
- weight, neighborhood, veil (sounds like "a")

To add a suffix to words ending with the letter "e," first determine if the "e" is silent. If it is, the "e" will be kept if the added suffix begins with a consonant. If the suffix begins with a vowel, the "e" is dropped. For example:
- age becomes ageless (keep the "e")
- age becomes aging (drop the "e")
An exception to this rule occurs when the word ends in "ce" or "ge" and the suffix "able" or "ous" is added; these words will retain the letter "e." The following are examples:
- courage becomes courageous
- notice becomes noticeable

<u>Words ending with "is," and "ize"</u>
A small number of words end with "ise." Most of the words in the English language

with the same sound end in "ize." The following are examples:

- advertise, advise, arise, chastise, circumcise, and comprise
- compromise, demise, despise, devise, disguise, enterprise, excise, and exercise
- franchise, improvise, incise, merchandise, premise, reprise, and revise
- supervise, surmise, surprise, and televise

Words that end with "ize" include the following:

- accessorize, agonize, authorize, and brutalize
- capitalize, caramelize, categorize, civilize, and demonize
- downsize, empathize, euthanize, idolize, and immunize
- legalize, metabolize, mobilize, organize, and ostracize
- plagiarize, privatize, utilize, and visualize

(Note that some words may technically be spelled with "ise," especially in British English, but it is more common to use "ize." Examples include symbolize/symbolise, and baptize/baptise.)

Words ending with "ceed," "sede," and "cede"
There are only three words that end with "ceed" in the English language: exceed, proceed, and succeed. There is only one word that ends with "sede," and that word is supersede. Many other words (that sound like "sede") end with "cede." The following are examples:

- concede, recede, precede, and supercede

Words ending in "able" or "ible"
For words ending in "able" or "ible," there are no hardfast rules. The following are examples:

- adjustable, unbeatable, collectable, deliverable, and likeable
- edible, compatible, feasible, sensible, and credible

There are more words ending in "able" than "ible;" this is useful to know if guessing is necessary.

Words ending in "ance" and "ence"
The suffixes "ence," "ency," and "ent" are used in the following cases:

- the suffix is preceded by the letter "c" but sounds like "s" – innocence
- the suffix is preceded by the letter "g" but sounds like "j" – intelligence, negligence

The suffixes "ance," "ancy," and "ant" are used in the following cases:

- the suffix is preceded by the letter "c" but sounds like "k" – significant, vacant
- the suffix is preceded by the letter "g" with a hard sound - elegant, extravagance

If the suffix is preceded by other letters, there are no steadfast rules. For example: finance, elegance, and defendant use the letter "a," while respondent, competence, and excellent use the letter "e."

Words ending "tion," "sion," and "cian"
Words ending in "tion," "sion," and "cian" all sound like "shun" or "zhun." There are no rules for which ending is used for words. The following are examples:

- action, agitation, caution, fiction, nation, and motion
- admission, expression, mansion, permission, and television
- electrician, magician, musician, optician, and physician (note that these words tend to describe occupations)

- 80 -

Words with the "ai" or "ia" combination

When deciding if "ai" or "ia" is correct, the combination of "ai" usually sounds like one vowel sound, as in "Britain," while the vowels in "ia" are pronounced separately, as in "guardian." The following are examples:

- captain, certain, faint, hair, malaise, and praise ("ai" makes one sound)
- bacteria, beneficiary, diamond, humiliation, and nuptial ("ia" makes two sounds)

Plural forms of nouns

Nouns ending in ch, sh, s, x, or z

When a noun ends in the letters ch, sh, s, x, or z, an es instead of a singular s is added to the end of the word to make it plural. The following are examples:

- church becomes churches
- bush becomes bushes
- bass becomes basses
- mix becomes mixes
- buzz becomes buzzes

This is the rule with proper names as well; the Ross family would become the Rosses.

Nouns ending in y or ay/ey/iy/oy/uy

If a noun ends with a consonant and y, the plural is formed by replacing the *y* with *ies*. For example, *fly* becomes *flies* and *puppy* becomes *puppies*.
If a noun ends with a vowel and *y*, the plural is formed by adding an *s*. For example, *alley* becomes *alleys* and *boy* becomes *boys*.

Nouns ending in f or fe

Most nouns ending in f or fe are pluralized by replacing the f with v and adding es. The following are examples:

- knife becomes knives; self becomes selves; wolf becomes wolves.

An exception to this rule is the word roof; roof becomes roofs.

Nouns ending in o

Most nouns ending with a consonant and o are pluralized by adding es. The following are examples:

- hero becomes heroes; tornado becomes tornadoes; potato becomes potatoes

Most nouns ending with a vowel and o are pluralized by adding s. The following are examples:

- portfolio becomes portfolios; radio becomes radios; shoe becomes shoes.

An exception to these rules is seen with musical terms ending in o. These words are pluralized by adding s even if they end in a consonant and o. The following are examples:
soprano becomes sopranos; banjo becomes banjos; piano becomes pianos.

Exceptions to the rules of plurals

Some words do not fall into any specific category for making the singular form plural. They are irregular. Certain words become plural by changing the vowels within the word. The following are examples:

- woman becomes women; goose becomes geese; foot becomes feet

Some words become completely different words in the plural form. The following are examples:

- mouse becomes mice; fungus becomes fungi; alumnus becomes alumni

Some words are the same in both the singular and plural forms. The following are examples:

- Salmon, species, and deer are all the same whether singular or plural.

Plural forms of letters, numbers, symbols, and compound nouns with hyphens

Letters and numbers become plural by adding an apostrophe and s. The following are examples:

- The L's are the people whose names begin with the letter L.
- They broke the teams down into groups of 3's.
- The sorority girls were all KD's.

A compound noun is a noun that is comprised of two or more words; they can be written with hyphens. For example, mother-in-law or court-martial are compound nouns. To make them plural, an s or es is added to the main word. The following are examples: mother-in-law becomes mothers-in-law; court-martial becomes court-martials.

Capitalization

Sentences, poetry, formal statements, and calendar terms
The first word of every sentence is capitalized. When citing poetry, the first word in every line should be capitalized. For example, the beginning of Annabel Lee by Edgar Allan Poe would be quoted as follows:
It was many and many a year ago,
In a kingdom by the sea....
The first word in formal statements or direct quotations should be capitalized. The following is an example:
"For immediate release: the company has declared bankruptcy."
Calendar terms to be capitalized include the days of the week (Friday, etc.), months of the year (December, etc.), and holidays (Halloween, Easter, etc.).

Proper names, seasons, literary works, and family names
Proper names and titles are capitalized, as are military ranks. The following are examples:

- Jack Carter, Ph.D.
- Princess of Wales
- Senator Max Baucus
- Lieutenant Kathy Johnson

The names of seasons (spring, summer, fall, and winter) are not capitalized unless they are part of a literary quote in which they are capitalized. In literary works such as books, chapters, plays, poems, and articles, the main words are capitalized. Articles (and, the, etc.) are usually not capitalized unless they are the first word. The following provides examples:
The King and I is my favorite play; I also like the book A Time to Kill.
Notice that these are also underlined. Family titles such as uncle or cousin are not capitalized unless they are part of a proper noun or a title. The following provides examples:
Uncle Billy is coming for dinner; he is not bringing his cousin Steve.

Geography
The names of geographical places (states, countries, oceans, etc.) should be capitalized. The following provides examples:

- Houston, Texas is by the Gulf of Mexico; the Rio Grande flows through the western part of the state.

When using directions such as north, south, east, or west, they should be capitalized if they are referring to particular regions. They should not be capitalized if referring to parts of states or when they are points on the compass. The following are examples:

- Louisiana is part of the South.
- I live in western Kentucky.

- John's compass indicated that we are traveling east.

The names of city streets, memorials, or parks should be capitalized if they are used as proper nouns. The following are examples:
- Rose walks past the Lincoln Memorial every day.
- You live on Oak Avenue; that's a nice avenue.

Notice that "avenue" is not capitalized the second time.

History and religion

Historical events such as wars, battles, and treaties and historical documents are capitalized: World War II, Magna Carta, and Battle of Gettysburg. The names of organized associations are also capitalized: Republican Party, United Way, and Sigma Chi.

Words that indicate where something or someone originated are capitalized. The following provides examples:

He is a German from Germany; he also likes German sausage.

The names of religions are capitalized: Catholic Church, Buddhism, and Islam. The names of gods and deities are also capitalized: Messiah, Brahma, and Allah. In some Christian writings, the pronoun "he" is capitalized when it refers to God or Jesus Christ.

Period

A period (.) is put at the end of a declarative sentence, a sentence that states a fact or idea. The following sentence is an example:

(1) The cat crossed the street.

A period is also at the end of an imperative sentence, which is a type of command. The following is an example:

(1) Bring the bag over here.

A period follows an indirect question. The following is an example:

(1) She wants to know how the game works.

A period is also used for abbreviations, such as Ms., B.C., or Capt. for Captain. A group of periods is called an ellipsis. These are used when quoted material is only partially copied. An ellipsis contains three periods at the beginning of a sentence, three periods in the middle of a sentence, or four periods at the end of a sentence. The following sentence provides an example:

"...Then he picked up the groceries...paid for them...later he went home...."

Comma

A comma (,) has many uses. Things in a list should be separated by commas. The following is an example:

(1) They saw John, Mary, and Drew at the game.

In a complex sentence, the clauses are separated by commas. If both clauses are independent, remove the comma and the connecting word and the sentences should be able to stand alone. The following is an example:

(1) It was August, and it was hot.

Both "It was August" and "It was hot" can stand alone as sentences.

A comma is used to set off the words yes and no. A comma will be used to offset a clause or phrase. The following is an example:

(1) Yes, I met Paul yesterday.

A comma separates a city and state (Seattle, Washington) and is used when writing dates (November 1, 1999). A greeting in an informal letter is set off by a comma (Dear Joseph,). A comma is also used when words are quoted. The following is an example:

"One time," I said, "I found fifty dollars."

Colon

The colon (:) is similar to a comma or semicolon but is used when a longer pause is necessary between the phrases.

It can sometimes indicate words that need to be emphasized in the sentence. The following is an example:

> (1) When you go to the airport, remember: don't forget your ticket!

A colon is used when writing time (4:25 a.m.) or after a greeting in a formal letter (Dear Sir:). A colon can be used to set off quotes; in that instance, the quote is usually capitalized. The following is an example:

> (1) Margaret loved to quote Shakespeare: "To thine own self be true."

Colons are also used by playwrights when writing dialogue.

Semicolon

A semicolon (;) separates two independent clauses if they are not joined by a connective conjunction. The following is an example:

> (1) Abby reads books; she likes to watch television too.

The two phrases could have been joined by the word "and" but a semicolon is used instead. A semicolon is also used to join two phrases connected by a conjunctive adverb. Examples of conjunctive adverbs include therefore, however, thus, and furthermore.

The following is an example:

> (1) It was raining; therefore, the baseball game was cancelled.

A semicolon can also be used if a sentence contains many commas. The following is an example:

They were wet, cold, and tired; but they were still in very good spirits.

Hyphen

A hyphen (-) is used to divide a word that will not fit on the line of the sentence. The word should be divided between syllables. The following is an example:

> (1) Leslie and Mark want to attend college at the

University of Southern Alabama.

Numbers from twenty-one to ninety-nine are written with hyphens (sixty-seven or thirty-five). Fractions that are used as adjectives are also written with hyphens (two-fifths of the senior class).

If a word begins with any of the following prefixes, a hyphen is used: great, trans, all, ex, and self. Examples include great-grandmother, self-aware, and ex-wife. If a prefix precludes a proper noun or adjective, a hyphen is used, such as with "mid-January."

A hyphen can be used to distinguish words that have different meanings but the same spelling, such as "re-sign" a contract versus "resign" from a job.

Parentheses

Parentheses ( ) are used in pairs to enclose words or phrases that supplement the main sentence. They are placed in the middle and can interrupt the flow. The following is an example:

Brian went to Los Angeles (his favorite city) and went surfing.

If the statement in the parentheses is an entire sentence that can stand on its own, it does not need a separate punctuation mark, unless it is a question; then it would need a question mark. The following is an example:

> (1) I saw Susan at the new grocery store (have you been there?) and she asked about you.

Parentheses can also be used to list items. The following is an example:

For the party we need (1) cake, (2) food, and (3) music.

Quotation mark

A pair of quotation marks ("") encloses quoted words or phrases whether the quoted section states what someone said or is a formal quote from a copyrighted work. The following are examples:

(1) Amy said, "I have a new house."

(2) In the novel Jane Eyre, Charlotte Bronte wrote, "Reader, I married him."

Quotes are also used for titles of short articles, poems, chapters, songs, or essays. When using slang terms, quotes can be used. The following is an example:

(1) Charlie considers himself a serious "gamer" and has an Xbox.

If a quote is used within a quote, use a single quotation mark. The following is an example:

(1) Mr. Turner said, "Edward R. Murrow used to say, 'Good night, and good luck.'"

Quotation marks are almost always placed after the final punctuation mark (period, question mark, etc.) in a sentence.

Bracket

Brackets ([ ]) can be used to add explanatory or descriptive information to a sentence. The following is an example:

(1) Jay's Place [the new coffee shop] has great espresso.

When quoting material, it is sometimes necessary to change a word or pronoun to fit the structure of the new sentence. Brackets will be used around the new word to show that it is different from the original. For example, "Jessica noted that her shirt is pink" could be replaced with the following:

(1) Jessica noted that "[my] shirt is pink."

If a quoted word is misspelled, the word sic (which literally means "that's how it was") may be added within brackets. The following is an example:

(1) "Jesse is the best mathematician [sic] in the club."

Brackets can be complicated and should be used sparingly. Parentheses are more common.

Apostrophe

An apostrophe (') and the letter s show possession. They are added after a singular noun. The following is an example:

(1) Susie's car, Steve's idea, and Carl's money were all a part of the plan.

If the possessive is to be made from a word that already ends in the letter s, only an apostrophe will be added to avoid too many s sounds. The following is an example:

(1) Carlos' hat is over there.

A plural noun can be made possessive: The children's bookstore is great. Follow the rule of s with plural nouns. For example, if more than one boy had a basketball, they would be the boys' basketballs.

Apostrophes are used with words, letters, or numbers that do not have a specific rule for plurals. The following is an example:

(1) The t's need to be crossed.

(2) They went to school in groups of 3's.

A contraction (can't or won't) uses an apostrophe. Dates can be shortened by using apostrophes, such as "born in '08."

Question mark, exclamation mark, and dash

The question mark (?) is used at the end of a sentence that asks a direct question. The following is an example:

(1) How many hours have you been gone?

In the case of an informal, polite request, a period may be used. The following is an example:

(1) Will you please pass the salt.

An exclamation mark (!) is used when the sentence expresses extreme emotion. The following is an example:

(1) I passed my final exam!

A dash (–) is used in a sentence when the context or idea suddenly changes pace. It

- 85 -

can also indicate an interruption. The following is an example:

> (1) Kate chose the red dress – you thought she'd get the black one – and then went to the dance.

Slash

The slash (/) is used to indicate that the reader has a choice between words. It can be used in some instances in place of the word or. The following is an example:

> (1) It was a pass/fail type of test.

Slashes are sometimes used to illustrate gender indifference, such as with his/her, he/she, or him/her. If used in this way, there are no spaces before and after the slash.

When slashes are used in quoted material, usually poetry, there are spaces before and after the slash. The following is an example:

"Shall I compare thee to a summer's day? / Thou art more lovely and more temperate..."

Commonly misspelled words

accidentally	conceive	finally	momentous
accommodate	congratulations	forehead	mortgage
accompanied	conqueror	foreign	neither
accompany	conscious	foreign	nickel
achieved	coolly	foremost	niece
acknowledgment	correspondent	forfeit	ninety
across	courtesy	ghost	noticeable
address	curiosity	glamorous	notoriety
aggravate	cylinder	government	obedience
aisle	deceive	grammar	obstacle
ancient	deference	grateful	occasion
anxiety	deferred	grief	occurrence
apparently	definite	grievous	omitted
appearance	describe	handkerchief	operate
arctic	desirable	harass	optimistic
argument	desperate	hoping	organization
arrangement	develop	hurriedly	outrageous
attendance	diphtheria	hygiene	pageant
auxiliary	disappear	hypocrisy	pamphlet
awkward	disappoint	imminent	parallel
bachelor	disastrous	incidentally	parliament
barbarian	discipline	incredible	permissible
beggar	discussion	independent	perseverance
beneficiary	disease	indigestible	persuade
biscuit	dissatisfied	inevitable	physically
brilliant	dissipate	innocence	physician
business	drudgery	intelligible	possess
cafeteria	ecstasy	intentionally	possibly
calendar	efficient	intercede	practically
campaign	eighth	interest	prairie
candidate	eligible	irresistible	preceding
ceiling	embarrass	judgment	prejudice
cemetery	emphasize	legitimate	prevalent
changeable	especially	liable	professor
changing	exaggerate	library	pronunciation
characteristic	exceed	likelihood	pronunciation
chauffeur	exhaust	literature	propeller
colonel	exhilaration	maintenance	protein
column	existence	maneuver	psychiatrist
commit	explanation	manual	psychology
committee	extraordinary	mathematics	quantity
comparative	familiar	mattress	questionnaire
compel	fascinate	miniature	rally
competent	February	mischievous	recede
competition	fiery	misspell	receive

- 87 -

Commonly misspelled words

recognize
recommend
referral
referred
relieve
religious
resistance
restaurant
rhetoric
rhythm
ridiculous
sacrilegious
salary
scarcely
schedule
secretary
sentinel
separate
severely
sheriff
shriek
similar
soliloquy
sophomore
species
strenuous
studying
suffrage
supersede
suppress
surprise
symmetry
temperament
temperature
tendency
tournament
tragedy
transferred
truly
twelfth
tyranny
recognize
recommend
referral
referred

unanimous
unpleasant
usage
vacuum
valuable
vengeance
vigilance
villain
Wednesday
weird
wholly
yolk

Structure

Beginning a sentence with the words and or but

The conjunctions and and but should generally be used to join two parts of a sentence. However, some writers may feel the need to begin a sentence with one of these conjunctions. While it is a practice that is frowned upon for formal writing, it can be acceptable in less formal narratives and stories. Before beginning a sentence with and or but, the writer should carefully consider whether the use of the conjunction would alter the meaning of the sentence. Can the sentence function without the addition of the conjunction? Also consider whether it would be better to connect the sentence to the previous sentence rather than allow it to stand alone.

Types of sentences

For a sentence to be complete, it must have a subject and a verb or predicate. A complete sentence will express a complete thought, otherwise it is known as a fragment. An example of a fragment is: "..as the clock struck midnight." A complete sentence would be: "As the clock struck midnight, she ran home." The types of sentences are declarative, imperative, interrogative, and exclamatory.
A declarative sentence states a fact and ends with a period. The following is an example:

(1) The football game starts at seven o'clock.

An imperative sentence tells someone to do something and ends with a period. The following is an example:

(1) Go to the store and buy milk.

An interrogative sentence asks a question and ends with a question mark. The following is an example:

(1) Are you going to the game on Friday?

An exclamatory sentence shows strong emotion and ends with an exclamation point. The following is an example:
I can't believe we won the game!

Modes of sentence patterns

Sentence patterns fall into five common modes with some exceptions. They are:

- Subject + linking verb + subject complement
- Subject + transitive verb + direct object
- Subject + transitive verb + indirect object + direct object
- Subject + transitive verb + direct object + object complement
- Subject + intransitive verb

Common exceptions to these patterns are questions and commands, sentences with delayed subjects, and passive transformations. Writers sometimes use the passive voice when the active voice would be more appropriate.

Transitions

Transitions are bridges between what has been read and what is about to be read. Transitions smooth the reader's path between sentences and inform the reader of major connections to new ideas forthcoming in the text. Transitional phrases should be used with care, selecting the appropriate phrase for a transition. Tone is another important consideration in using transitional phrases, varying the tone for different audiences. For example, in a scholarly essay, "in summary" would be preferable to the more informal "in short."
When working with transitional words and phrases, writers usually find a natural flow that indicates when a transition is needed. In reading a draft of the text, it

should become apparent where the flow is uneven or rough. At this point, the writer can add transitional elements during the revision process. Revising can also afford an opportunity to delete transitional devices that seem heavy handed or unnecessary.

Transitional words and phrases are used to transition between paragraphs and also to transition within a single paragraph. Transitions assist the flow of ideas and help to unify an essay. A writer can use certain words to indicate that an example or summary is being presented. The following phrases, among others, can be used as this type of transition: *as a result, as I have said, for example, for instance, in any case, in any event, in brief, in conclusion, in fact, in other words, in short, on the whole,* and *to sum it up.*

Transitional words

Link similar ideas

Transitional words and phrases are used to transition between paragraphs and also to transition within a single paragraph. Transitions assist the flow of ideas and help to unify an essay. When a writer links ideas that are similar in nature, there are a variety of words and phrases he or she can choose, including but not limited to: *also, and, another, besides, equally important, further, furthermore, in addition, likewise, too, similarly, nor, of course,* and *for instance.*

Link dissimilar or contradictory ideas

Transitional words and phrases are used to transition between paragraphs and also to transition within a single paragraph. Transitions assist the flow of ideas and help to unify an essay. Writers can link contradictory ideas in an essay by using, among others, the following words and phrases: *although, and yet, even if, conversely, but, however, otherwise, still, yet, instead, in spite of, nevertheless, on the contrary,* and *on the other hand.*

Indicate cause, purpose, or result

Transitional words and phrases are used to transition between paragraphs and also to transition within a single paragraph. Transitions assist the flow of ideas and help to unify an essay. Writers may need to indicate that one thing is the cause, purpose, or result of another thing. To show this relationship, writers can use, among others, the following linking words and phrases: *as, as a result, because, consequently, hence, for, for this reason, since, so, then, thus,* and *therefore.*

Indicate time or position

Transitional words and phrases are used to transition between paragraphs and also to transition within a single paragraph. Transitions assist the flow of ideas and help to unify an essay. Certain words can be used to indicate the time and position of one thing in relation to another. Writers can use, for example, the following terms to create a timeline of events in an essay: *above, across, afterward, before, beyond, eventually, meanwhile, next, presently, around, at once, at the present time, finally, first, here, second, thereafter,* and *upon.* These words can show the order or placement of items or ideas in an essay.

Commas

Abbreviations, interjections, and direct addresses

Abbreviations, interjections, and direct addresses are all types of sentence interruptions. An interruption is any word or phrase that stops the flow of a sentence. Interruptions should be set off by commas. Abbreviations such as Jr. or Ph.D. must be set off by commas. (*Harry Langford, Ph.D., will be hosting the event.*) Interjections are exclamations that lack grammatical connection to a sentence. A comma should be inserted before and after an interjection. (*Oh, you must be joking.*) A direct address occurs when the writer speaks directly to another person.

The term used to address the person must be set off by commas. (*No, Mother, I will not lower my voice.*)

Geographical references, transitional words and phrases, and parenthetical words and phrases

Geographical references, transitional words and phrases, and parenthetical words and phrases are all types of sentence interruptions. An interruption is any word or phrase that stops the flow of a sentence. Interruptions should be set off by commas. Geographical references include the names of a city within a state or a specific street address. (*I will visit Detroit, Michigan, in September.*) As in this example, a comma should be placed after the name of the city and another comma should be placed after the name of the state if the sentence continues. Transitional words and phrases include sayings such as *on the other hand, contrary to popular belief*, and *nevertheless*. These expressions must be set off from the rest of the sentence with commas. Parenthetical words and phrases are similar to transitional phrases and must also be set off from the rest of the sentence with commas.

Parallel structure in a sentence

Parallel sentence structure refers to the use of similar word patterns to show that each idea in a sentence has equal importance. Parallel structure can involve single words, phrases, or clauses within a sentence. In the sentence *Susan enjoys painting, singing, and reading*, the words *painting, singing*, and *reading* all end with *-ing*, which creates a parallel structure. The conjunctions and and or usually signal the need for parallel structure.

Sentence structure

The four major types of sentence structure are:

- Simple sentences: Simple sentences have one independent clause with no subordinate clauses. A simple sentence may contain compound elements—a compound subject, verb, or object, for example—but does not contain more than one full sentence pattern.
- Compound sentences: Compound sentences are composed of two or more independent clauses with no subordinate clauses. The independent clauses are usually joined with a comma and a coordinating conjunction or with a semicolon.
- Complex sentences: A complex sentence is composed of one independent clause with one or more dependent clauses.
- Compound-complex sentences: A compound-complex sentence contains at least two independent clauses and at least one subordinate clause. Sometimes they contain two full sentence patterns that can stand alone. When each independent clause contains a subordinate clause, this makes the sentence both compound and complex.

Paragraph length

The reader's comfort level is paragraphs of between 100 and 200 words. Shorter paragraphs cause too much starting and stopping, and give a choppy effect. Paragraphs that are too long often test the attention span of the reader. Two notable exceptions to this rule exist. In scientific or scholarly papers, longer paragraphs suggest seriousness and depth. In journalistic writing, constraints are placed on paragraph size by the narrow columns in a newspaper format. The first and last paragraphs of a text will usually be the introduction and conclusion. These special-purpose paragraphs are likely to be shorter than paragraphs in the body of the work. Paragraphs in the body of the essay follow the subject's outline; one paragraph per point in short essays and a group of paragraphs per point in longer ones work. Some ideas require more development than others do, so it is good for a writer to remain flexible. A too-long paragraph may be divided, and shorter ones may be combined.

Coherent paragraphs

A smooth flow of sentences and paragraphs without gaps, shifts, or bumps leads to paragraph coherence. Ties between old and new information can be smoothed by several strategies:

- Linking ideas clearly, from the topic sentence to the body of the paragraph, is essential for a smooth transition. The topic sentence states the main point, and this should be followed by specific details, examples, and illustrations that support the topic sentence. The support may be direct or indirect. In indirect support, the illustrations and examples may support a sentence that in turn supports the topic directly.
- The repetition of key words adds coherence to a paragraph. To avoid dull language, variations of the key words may be used.
- Parallel structures are often used within sentences to emphasize the similarity of ideas and connect sentences giving similar information.
- Maintaining a consistent verb tense throughout the paragraph helps. Shifting tenses affects the smooth flow of words and can disrupt the coherence of the paragraph.

Main point of a paragraph

A paragraph should be unified around a main point. A good topic sentence summarizes the paragraph's main point. A topic sentence is more general than subsequent supporting sentences are. Sometime the topic sentence will be used to close the paragraph if earlier sentences give a clear indication of the direction of the paragraph. Sticking to the main point means deleting or omitting unnecessary sentences that do not advance the main point.

The main point of a paragraph deserves adequate development, which usually means a substantial paragraph. A paragraph of two or three sentences often does not develop a point well enough, particularly if the point is a strong supporting argument of the thesis. An occasional short paragraph is fine, particularly if it is used as a transitional device. A choppy appearance should be avoided.

Examining paragraphs and sentences

Paragraphs are a key structural unit of prose used to break up long stretches of words into more manageable subsets and to indicate a shift in topics or focus. Each paragraph may be examined by identifying the main point of the section and ensuring that every sentence supports or relates to the main theme. Paragraphs may be checked to make sure the organization used in each is appropriate and that the number of sentences is adequate to develop the topic.

Sentences are the building blocks of the written word, and they can be varied by paying attention to sentence length, sentence structure, and sentence openings. These elements should be varied so that writing does not seem boring, repetitive, or choppy. A careful analysis of a piece of writing will expose these stylistic problems, and they can be corrected before the final draft is written. Varying sentence structure and length can make writing more inviting and appealing to a reader.

Essay paragraph types

Explanation: gives examples, facts, and details
Compare and contrast: discusses how things are similar or different
Chronological: arranged according to timing
Spatial: arranged according to location
Emphasis: arranged in order of importance
Cause and effect: arranged from effect to cause or cause to effect
Problem/solution: arranged according to issues and solutions
Topical: arranged according to topics discussed

Simple sentence

A simple sentence is an independent clause that contains a complete subject and a complete predicate. Simple sentences can be very short or long; the length does not indicate the complexity of the sentence. The subject may be singular or compound (more than one subject). The predicate may also be singular or compound. The following are examples:

- Judy watered the lawn. (singular subject, singular predicate)
- Judy and Alan watered the lawn. (compound subject, Judy and Alan)
- Judy watered the lawn and planted flowers. (compound predicate, watered and planted)
- Judy and Alan watered the lawn and planted flowers. (compound subject and predicate)

Compound sentence

A compound sentence consists or two or more simple sentences joined together by a conjunction. Conjunctions can also be called coordinators and include the following: and, but, or, nor, for, yet, and so. A comma is written after the simple sentence and before the conjunction. The following is an example:

- I woke up at dawn, so I went outside to watch the sunrise.

A way to identify a compound sentence is to remove the conjunction and see if the two clauses can stand alone as simple sentences. In this case, "I woke up at dawn" and "I went outside to watch the sunset" can be independent; therefore, the sentence is a compound sentence.

Complex sentence

A complex sentence is comprised of an independent clause and one or more dependent clauses. The independent clause can exist alone as a sentence while a dependent clause needs to be grouped with an independent clause even though it has its own subject and verb. A dependent clause cannot exist alone as a sentence. Dependent clauses are linked to the independent clause with conjunctions, such as after, although, as, because, before, that, when, which, and while. The following are examples:

- Although he had the flu, Harry went to work.
- Marcia got married after she finished college.

Notice that the clause can appear before or after the independent phrase.

Reading Test

DIRECTIONS: The reading practice test you are about to take is multiple-choice with only one correct answer per question. Read each test item and circle your answer on the answer sheet below. When you have completed the practice test, you may check your answers with those on the answer key that follows the test.

Answer Sheet

1.	a	b	c	d		25.	a	b	c	d
2.	a	b	c	d		26.	a	b	c	d
3.	a	b	c	d		27.	a	b	c	d
4.	a	b	c	d		28.	a	b	c	d
5.	a	b	c	d		29.	a	b	c	d
6.	a	b	c	d		30.	a	b	c	d
7.	a	b	c	d		31.	a	b	c	d
8.	a	b	c	d		32.	a	b	c	d
9.	a	b	c	d		33.	a	b	c	d
10.	a	b	c	d		34.	a	b	c	d
11.	a	b	c	d		35.	a	b	c	d
12.	a	b	c	d		36.	a	b	c	d
13.	a	b	c	d		37.	a	b	c	d
14.	a	b	c	d		38.	a	b	c	d
15.	a	b	c	d		39.	a	b	c	d
16.	a	b	c	d		40.	a	b	c	d
17.	a	b	c	d		41.	a	b	c	d
18.	a	b	c	d		42.	a	b	c	d
19.	a	b	c	d		43.	a	b	c	d
20.	a	b	c	d		44.	a	b	c	d
21.	a	b	c	d		45.	a	b	c	d
22.	a	b	c	d		46.	a	b	c	d
23.	a	b	c	d		47.	a	b	c	d
24.	a	b	c	d		48.	a	b	c	d

1. Adelaide attempted to <u>assuage</u> her guilt over the piece of cheesecake by limiting herself to salads the following day. Which of the following is the definition for the underlined word in the sentence above?

    a. increase
    b. support
    c. appease
    d. conceal

2. Hilaire's professor instructed him to improve the word choice in his papers. As the professor noted, Hilaire's ideas are good, but he relies too heavily on simple expressions when a more complex word would be appropriate. Which of the following resources will be most useful to Hilaire in this case?

    a. Roget's Thesaurus
    b. Oxford Latin Dictionary
    c. Encyclopedia Britannica
    d. Webster's Dictionary

Questions 3 – 5 pertain to the following:

    The Dewey Decimal Classes
    000 Computer science, information, and general works
    100 Philosophy and psychology
    200 Religion
    300 Social sciences
    400 Languages
    500 Science and mathematics
    600 Technical and applied science
    700 Arts and recreation
    800 Literature
    900 History, geography, and biography

3. Lise is doing a research project on the various psychological theories that Sigmund Freud developed and on the modern response to those theories. She is not sure where to begin, so she consults the chart of Dewey Decimal Classes. To which section of the library should she go to begin looking for research material?

    a. 100
    b. 200
    c. 300
    d. 900

4. During her research, Lise discovers that Freud's theory of the Oedipal complex was based on ancient Greek mythology that was made famous by Sophocles' play *Oedipus Rex*. To which section of the library should she go if she is interested in reading the play?

    a. 300
    b. 400
    c. 800
    d. 900

5. Also during her research, Lise learns about Freud's Jewish background, and she decides to compare Freud's theories to traditional Judaism. To which section of the library should she go for more information on this subject?
   a. 100
   b. 200
   c. 800
   d. 900

6. Chapter 15: Roman Emperors in the First Century
   - Tiberius, 14-37 AD
   - Nero, 54-68 AD
   - Domitian, 81-96 AD
   - Hadrian, 117-138 AD

Analyze the headings above. Which of the following does not belong?
   a. Tiberius, 14-37 AD
   b. Nero, 54-68 AD
   c. Domitian, 81-96 AD
   d. Hadrian, 117-138 AD

7. Although his friends believed him to be enjoying a lavish lifestyle in the large family estate he had inherited, Enzo was in reality impecunious.
Which of the following is the definition for the underlined word in the sentence above?
   a. Penniless
   b. Unfortunate
   c. Emotional
   d. Commanding

8. Follow the numbered instructions to transform the starting word into a different word.
   1. Start with the word ESOTERIC
   2. Remove both instances of the letter E from the word
   3. Remove the letter I from the word
   4. Move the letter T from the middle of the word to the end of the word
   5. Remove the letter C from the word

What new word has been spelled?
   a. SECT
   b. SORT
   c. SORE
   d. TORE

Question 9 and 10 pertains to the chart below, which reflects the enrollment and the income for a small community college.

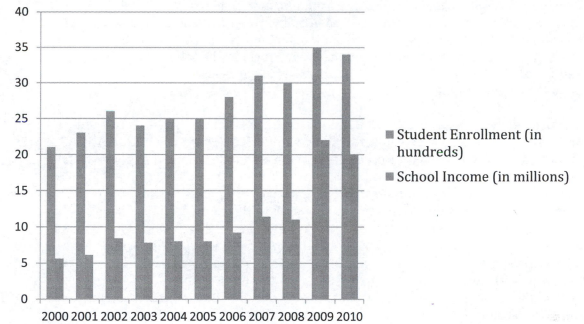

9. Based on the chart, approximately how many students attended the community college in the year 2001?
    a. 2100
    b. 2300
    c. 2500
    d. 2700

10. In order to offset costs, the college administration decided to increase enrollment costs. Reviewing the chart above, during which year is it most likely that the college raised the cost of enrollment?
    a. 2002
    b. 2007
    c. 2009
    d. 2010

11. The journalist, as part of his ongoing series of articles about the defendant accused of multiple murders, included a note that the defendant had written: "*No matter what they say I am not gilty [sic] of the crime.*" Which of the following does the bracketed expression "*sic*" indicate?
    a. An accidental misspelling in the sentence
    b. A grammatical error that the editor failed to catch
    c. An incorrect usage on the part of the original writer
    d. A point of emphasis that the journalist wants readers to see

Questions 12 – 15 are based on the passage below:
    The area known as the Bermuda Triangle has become such a part of popular culture that it can be difficult to separate fact from fiction. The interest first began when five Navy planes vanished in 1945, officially resulting from "causes or reasons unknown." The explanations about other accidents in the Triangle range from the

scientific to the supernatural. Researchers have never been able to find anything truly mysterious about what happens in the Bermuda Triangle, if there even is a Bermuda Triangle. What is more, one of the biggest challenges in considering the phenomenon is deciding how much area actually represents the Bermuda Triangle. Most consider the Triangle to stretch from Miami out to Puerto Rico and to include the island of Bermuda. Others expand the area to include all of the Caribbean islands and to extend eastward as far as the Azores, which are closer to Europe than they are to North America.

The problem with having a larger Bermuda Triangle is that it increases the odds of accidents. There is near-constant travel, by ship and by plane, across the Atlantic, and accidents are expected to occur. In fact, the Bermuda Triangle happens to fall within one of the busiest navigational regions in the world, and the reality of greater activity creates the possibility for more to go wrong. Shipping records suggest that there is not a greater-than-average loss of vessels within the Bermuda Triangle, and many researchers have argued that the reputation of the Triangle makes any accident seem out of the ordinary. In fact, most accidents fall within the expected margin of error. The increase in ships from East Asia no doubt contributes to an increase in accidents. And as for the story of the Navy planes that disappeared within the Triangle, many researchers now conclude that it was the result of mistakes on the part of the pilots who were flying into storm clouds and simply got lost.

12. Which of the following describes this type of writing?
   a. Narrative
   b. Persuasive
   c. Expository
   d. Technical

13. Which of the following sentences is most representative of a summary sentence for this passage?
   a. The problem with having a larger Bermuda Triangle is that it increases the odds of accidents.
   b. The area that is called the Bermuda Triangle happens to fall within one of the busiest navigational regions in the world, and the reality of greater activity creates the possibility for more to go wrong.
   c. One of the biggest challenges in considering the phenomenon is deciding how much area actually represents the Bermuda Triangle.
   d. Researchers have never been able to find anything truly mysterious about what happens in the Bermuda Triangle, if there even is a Bermuda Triangle.

14. With which of the following statements would the author most likely agree?
   a. There is no real mystery about the Bermuda Triangle because most events have reasonable explanations.
   b. Researchers are wrong to expand the focus of the Triangle to the Azores, because this increases the likelihood of accidents.
   c. The official statement of "causes or reasons unknown" in the loss of the Navy planes was a deliberate concealment from the Navy.
   d. Reducing the legends about the mysteries of the Bermuda Triangle will help to reduce the number of reported accidents or shipping losses in that region.

15. Which of the following represents an opinion statement on the part of the author?
   a. The problem with having a larger Bermuda Triangle is that it increases the odds of accidents.
   b. The area known as the Bermuda Triangle has become such a part of popular culture that it can be difficult to sort through the myth and locate the truth.
   c. The increase in ships from East Asia no doubt contributes to an increase in accidents.
   d. Most consider the Triangle to stretch from Miami to Puerto Rico and include the island of Bermuda.

16. *But I don't like the beach*, Judith complained. *All that sand. It gets in between my toes, in my swimsuit, and in my hair and eyes.* Martin suggested an alternative. *Then, let's go to the park instead.* The use of italics in the text above indicates which of the following?
   a. Dialogue
   b. Emphasis
   c. Thoughts
   d. Anger

17. The guide words at the top of a dictionary page are *intrauterine* and *invest*. Which of the following words is an entry on this page?
   a. Intransigent
   b. Introspection
   c. Investiture
   d. Intone

18. The public eagerness to <u>lionize</u> the charming actor after his string of popular films kept his managers busy concealing his shady background and questionable activities.
Which of the following is the definition for the underlined word in the sentence above?
   a. Criticize
   b. Sympathize with
   c. Betray
   d. Glorify

19. Ninette has celiac disease, which means that she cannot eat any product containing gluten. Gluten is a protein present in many grains such as wheat, rye, and barley. Because of her health condition, Ninette has to be careful about what she eats to avoid having an allergic reaction. She will be attending an all-day industry event, and she requested the menu in advance.
   - Breakfast: Fresh coffee or tea, scrambled eggs, bacon or sausage
   - Lunch: Spinach salad (dressing available on the side), roasted chicken, steamed rice
   - Cocktail Hour: Various beverages, fruit and cheese plate
   - Dinner: Spaghetti and sauce, tossed salad, garlic bread

During which of these meals should Ninette be careful to bring her own food?
   a. Breakfast
   b. Lunch
   c. Cocktail Hour
   d. Dinner

20. Chapter 2: Shakespeare Before He Was Famous
   - Family Background
   - Childhood Experiences
   - Education
   - Dramatic Works
   - Youthful Marriage to Anne Hathaway
   - Move to London

Analyze the headings above. Which of the following does not belong?
   a. Family Background
   b. Education
   c. Dramatic Works
   d. Youthful Marriage to Anne Hathaway

21. *Letter to the Editor:*

   I was disappointed by the August 12ᵗʰ article entitled *"How to Conserve Water."* While the author of the article, Neil Chambers, provided excellent tips, he overlooked the most obvious--Z 09` taking shorter showers. Mr. Chambers should consider the recent study by Dr. James Duncan on the subject, which examines the importance of shower length in reducing water use:
   - While water conservation options vary, the most effective might also be one of the simplest. Consumers who take shorter showers can reduce their water usage significantly each year. The standard shower head allows releases more than two gallons of water per minute. By cutting each shower short by only five minutes, consumers can save over twelve gallons of water.

Water conservationists applaud the newspaper's efforts to direct readers toward opportunities to conserve, but journalists should put a little more effort into research before sending their work to publication.

Which of the following explains the reason for the indentation in the passage above?
   a. A quote from another source
   b. A conversation between two authorities on a subject
   c. A quoted portion from a published article by the author of the letter
   d. A disputed claim from the author of the newspaper article

22. With most of the evidence being circumstantial, the defense attorney was successful in his attempt to <u>exculpate</u> his client before the jury. Which of the following is the definition for the underlined word in the sentence above?
   a. Dismiss
   b. Clear
   c. Condemn
   d. Forgive

Questions 23 – 25 pertain to the chart below:

NAME	COMPOSITION (PER 100)	WORLD LITERATURE (PER 100)	TECHNICAL WRITING (PER 100)	LINGUISTICS (PER 100)
TEXTBOOK-MANIA	$4500	$5150	$6000	$6500
TEXTBOOK CENTRAL	$4350	$5200	$6100	$6550
BOOKSTORE SUPPLY	$4675	$5000	$5950	$6475
UNIVERSITY TEXTBOOKS	$4600	$5000	$6100	$6650

Note: Shipping is free for all schools that order 100 textbooks or more.

23. A school needs to purchase 500 composition textbooks and 500 world literature textbooks. Which of the textbook suppliers can offer the lowest price?
    a. Textbook Mania
    b. Textbook Central
    c. Bookstore Supply
    d. University Textbooks

24. A school needs to purchase 1000 composition textbooks and 300 linguistics textbooks. Which of the textbook suppliers can offer the lowest price?
    a. Textbook Mania
    b. Textbook Central
    c. Bookstore Supply
    d. University Textbooks

25. A school needs to purchase 400 world literature textbooks and 200 technical writing textbooks. Which of the textbook suppliers can offer the lowest price?
    a. Textbook Mania
    b. Textbook Central
    c. Bookstore Supply
    d. University Textbooks

26. Given his fascination with all things nautical, Blaise could not pass up the opportunity to tour the reproduction 18th-century bark that was docked nearby. Based on the context of the passage above, which of the following is the definition of the underlined word?
    a. The outside surface of a tree
    b. A crisp order
    c. A piece of hard chocolate-coated candy
    d. A sailing vessel

27. A cruise brochure offers a variety of options for Mediterranean cruises. The brochure notes that the ships cruising the Mediterranean pull into the following cities:

- Venice, Italy
- Athens, Greece
- Barcelona, Spain
- Oslo, Norway
- Istanbul, Turkey

Which of these cities is out of place in the list above?
   a. Athens, Greece
   b. Barcelona, Spain
   c. Oslo, Norway
   d. Istanbul, Turkey

28. The same brochure provides customers with a list of cities in the United States from which the cruises depart:

- Baltimore, MD
- Boston, MA
- Charleston, SC
- Fort Lauderdale, FL
- _____
- Miami, FL

Consider the pattern in the list of cities above. Which of the following cities belongs in the blank?
   a. Tampa, FL
   b. Galveston, TX
   c. Norfolk, VA
   d. New York, NY

Starting Image

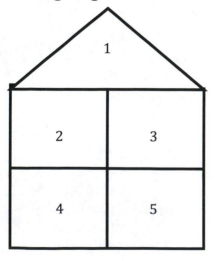

Start with the shape pictured above. Follow the directions to alter its appearance.

- Rotate section 1 90° clockwise and move it to the right side, against sections 3 and 5.
- Remove section 4.
- Move section 2 immediately above section 3.
- Swap section 2 and section 5.
- Remove section 5.
- Draw a circle around the shape, enclosing it completely.

29. Which of the following does the shape now look like?

a.

b.

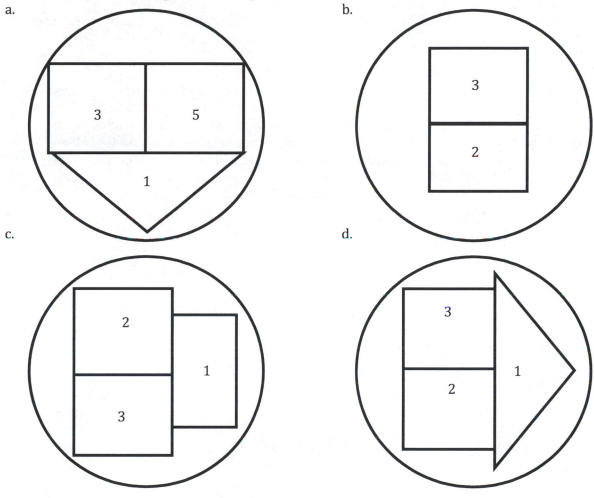

c.

d.

30. Anna is planning a trip to Bretagne, or Brittany, in the northwestern part of France. Since she knows very little about it, she is hoping to find the most up-to-date information with the widest variety of details about hiking trails, beaches, restaurants, and accommodations. Which of the following guides will be the best for her to review?
   a. *The Top Ten Places to Visit in Brittany*, published by a non-profit organization in Bretagne looking to draw tourism to the region (2010)
   b. *Getting to Know Nantes: Eating, Staying, and Sightseeing in Brittany's Largest City*, published by the French Ministry of Tourism (2009)
   c. *Hiking Through Bretagne: The Best Trails for Discovering Northwestern France*, published by a company that specializes in travel for those wanting to experience the outdoors (2008)
   d. *The Complete Guide to Brittany*, published by a travel book company that publishes guides for travel throughout Europe (2010)

Question 31 pertains to the following passage:

Despite the aura of challenge that surrounds the making of haggis, Scotland's most famous dish takes some time but is really quite simple to prepare. Start with a sheep's stomach. Wash well, and soak for several hours. At the end of soaking, turn the stomach inside out. Boil one sheep's heart and one sheep's liver for about half an hour. Drain water and chop finely. Chop two or three onions. Toast approximately one cup of oatmeal, and then mix the chopped heart, liver, and onions with several spices: salt, pepper, cayenne, and nutmeg, seasoned to your preference. Add approximately one cup of the broth of your choice. Stuff the sheep's stomach with the mixture, and tie carefully with cooking twine. Make sure the stomach is well sealed. Then, add the stomach to a pot of boiling water, reduce to a simmer, and cook for about three hours. Have a needle ready to prick the stomach gently when it swells--it's better to avoid a haggis explosion!

31. Which of the following best describes the purpose of the passage above?
   a. Narrative
   b. Descriptive
   c. Persuasive
   d. Expository

Question 32 & 33 pertains to the following image below:

207 HEATING AND AIR CONDITIONING

Furnace Cleaning

America's Heating Experts *204 Pine*	(222) 850-1730
Everby Furnace *483 Maple*	
Duct Cleaning	
Free Estimates	(222) 850-3592
Good Ducts, Ltd. *983 Pine*	(222) 850-4829
Hebert Air *758 Sycamore*	(222) 850-2938

Furnace Installation

Everby Furnace *483 Maple*	(222) 850-3592
Fields Furnace Installation *399 Elm*	(222) 850-5201
Young's Heating, Inc. *492 Elm*	(222) 850-2942

Furnace Parts and Supplies

Allen Heating & Air *394 Maple*	(222) 850-9605
US Best Furnace Supplies *603 Pine*	(222) 850-3333
Wilkes Heating Parts *4930 Oak Alley*	(222) 850-1940
Zimmer Furnace Parts *555 Cypress*	(222) 850-2919

Furnace Repair

Ferris Furnace *706 Willow*	
Free estimates for all work	(222) 850-4920
Perry Repairs *203 Sycamore*	(222) 850-3333
Thomas Refrigeration *849 Oak Alley*	
Call us 24 hours a day	(222) 850-9283
V&V Furnace Repair *492 Willow*	
Free estimates	
24-hour service	(222) 850-8694

Need Better Air?
Call Hebert!
Furnace Inspection
Duct Cleaning
Free Estimates For All Jobs
Call 222.850.2938

EVERYBY
The Best in Furnaces
- Installation
- Cleaning
- Free Estimates
(222) 850-3592

Allen Heating
Expert Furnace Installation
Business Discounts
222-850-9605

Furnace on the Fritz?
Give FERRIS Furnace a Call!
-Discounts for First-Time Clients-
(222) 850-4920

Thomas Refrigeration
24/7 Furnace Emergencies
222-850-9283

32. Edgar needs a new furnace, so he checks the telephone book for a local company that offers furnace installation services. He is also looking for a company that can provide cleaning after installation. Which of the following businesses should he call?

    a. Ferris Furnace
    b. Allen Heating & Air
    c. Everby Furnace
    d. Field's Furnace Installation

33. Pierre's furnace is not working properly, and he needs a repair service. Because it is already 11 PM, he is looking for a furnace repair business that offers 24-hour service. Since he does not know the extent of the damage, Pierre is also hoping for a free estimate. Which of the following businesses should he call?
- a. Ferris Furnace
- b. Perry Repairs
- c. Thomas Refrigeration
- d. V&V Furnace Repair

Questions 34 -36 pertain to the passage below:

As little as three years before her birth, few would have thought that the child born Princess Alexandrina Victoria would eventually become Britain's longest reigning monarch, Queen Victoria. She was born in 1819, the only child of Edward, Duke of Kent who was the fourth son of King George III. Ahead of Edward were three brothers, two of whom became king but none of whom produced a legitimate, surviving heir. King George's eldest son, who was eventually crowned King George IV, secretly married a Catholic commoner, Maria Fitzherbert, in 1783. The marriage was never officially recognized, and in 1795, George was persuaded to marry a distant cousin, Caroline of Brunswick. The marriage was bitter, and the two had only one daughter, Princess Charlotte Augusta. She was popular in England where her eventual reign was welcomed, but in a tragic event that shocked the nation, the princess and her stillborn son died in childbirth in 1817.

Realizing the precarious position of the British throne, the remaining sons of King George III were motivated to marry and produce an heir. The first in line was Prince Frederick, the Duke of York. Frederick married Princess Frederica Charlotte of Prussia, but the two had no children. After Prince Frederick was Prince William, the Duke of Clarence. William married Princess Adelaide of Saxe-Meiningen, and they had two sickly daughters, neither of whom survived infancy. Finally, Prince Edward, the Duke of Kent, threw his hat into the ring with his marriage to Princess Victoria of Saxe-Coburg-Saalfeld. The Duke of Kent died less than a year after his daughter's birth, but the surviving Duchess of Kent was not unaware of the future possibilities for her daughter. She took every precaution to ensure that the young Princess Victoria was healthy and safe throughout her childhood.

Princess Victoria's uncle William succeeded his brother George IV to become King William IV. The new king recognized his niece as his future heir, but he did not necessarily trust her mother. As a result, he was determined to survive until Victoria's eighteenth birthday to ensure that she could rule in her own right without the regency of the Duchess of Kent. The king's fervent prayers were answered: he died June 20, 1837, less than one month after Victoria turned eighteen. Though young and inexperienced, the young queen recognized the importance of her position and determined to rule fairly and wisely. The improbable princess who became queen ruled for more than sixty-three years, and her reign is considered to be one of the most important in British history.

34. Which of the following is a logical conclusion that can be drawn from the information in the passage above?
   a. Victoria's long reign provided the opportunity for her to bring balance to England and right the wrongs that had occurred during the reigns of her uncle's.
   b. It was the death of Princess Charlotte Augusta that motivated the remaining princes to marry and start families.
   c. The Duke of Kent had hoped for a son but was delighted with his good fortune in producing the surviving heir that his brothers had failed to produce.
   d. King William IV was unreasonably suspicious of the Duchess of Kent's motivations, as she cared only for her daughter's well-being.

35. What is the author's likely purpose in writing this passage about Queen Victoria?
   a. To persuade the reader to appreciate the accomplishments of Queen Victoria, especially when placed against the failures of her forebears.
   b. To introduce the historical impact of the Victorian Era by introducing to readers the queen who gave that era its name.
   c. To explain how small events in history placed an unlikely princess in line to become the queen of England.
   d. To indicate the role that King George III's many sons played in changing the history of England.

36. Based on the context of the passage, the reader can infer that this information is likely to appear in which of the following types of works?
   a. A scholarly paper
   b. A mystery
   c. A fictional story
   d. A biography

Question 37- 43 pertains to the following passage:

In 1603, Queen Elizabeth I of England died. She had never married and had no heir, so the throne passed to a distant relative: James Stuart, the son of Elizabeth's cousin and one-time rival for the throne, Mary, Queen of Scots. James was crowned King James I of England. At the time, he was also King James VI of Scotland, and the combination of roles would create a spirit of conflict that haunted the two nations for generations to come.

The conflict developed as a result of rising tensions among the people within the nations, as well as between them. Scholars in the 21st century are far too hasty in dismissing the role of religion in political disputes, but religion undoubtedly played a role in the problems that faced England and Scotland. By the time of James Stuart's succession to the English throne, the English people had firmly embraced the teachings of Protestant theology. Similarly, the Scottish Lowlands was decisively Protestant. In the Scottish Highlands, however, the clans retained their Catholic faith. James acknowledged the Church of England and still sanctioned the largely Protestant translation of the Bible that still bears his name.

James's son King Charles I proved himself to be less committed to the Protestant Church of England. Charles married the Catholic Princess Henrietta Maria of France, and there were suspicions among the English and the Lowland Scots that Charles was quietly a Catholic. Charles's own political troubles extended beyond religion in

- 107 -

this case, and he was beheaded in 1649. Eventually, his son King Charles II would be crowned, and this Charles is believed to have converted secretly to the Catholic Church. Charles II died without a legitimate heir, and his brother James ascended to the throne as King James II.

James was recognized to be a practicing Catholic, and his commitment to Catholicism would prove to be his downfall. James's wife Mary Beatrice lost a number of children during their infancy, and when she became pregnant again in 1687 the public became concerned. If James had a son, that son would undoubtedly be raised a Catholic, and the English people would not stand for this. Mary gave birth to a son, but the story quickly circulated that the royal child had died and the child named James's heir was a foundling smuggled in. James, his wife, and his infant son were forced to flee; and James's Protestant daughter Mary was crowned the queen.

In spite of a strong resemblance to the king, the young James was generally rejected among the English and the Lowland Scots, who referred to him as "the Pretender." But in the Highlands the Catholic princeling was welcomed. He inspired a group known as *Jacobites*, to reflect the Latin version of his name. His own son Charles, known affectionately as Bonnie Prince Charlie, would eventually raise an army and attempt to recapture what he believed to be his throne. The movement was soundly defeated at the Battle of Culloden in 1746, and England and Scotland have remained ostensibly Protestant ever since.

37. Which of the following sentences contains an opinion on the part of the author?
   a. James was recognized to be a practicing Catholic, and his commitment to Catholicism would prove to be his downfall.
   b. James' son King Charles I proved himself to be less committed to the Protestant Church of England.
   c. The movement was soundly defeated at the Battle of Culloden in 1746, and England and Scotland have remained ostensibly Protestant ever since.
   d. Scholars in the 21st century are far too hasty in dismissing the role of religion in political disputes, but religion undoubtedly played a role in the problems that faced England and Scotland.

38. Which of the following represents the best meaning of the word *foundling*, based on the context in the passage?
   a. Orphan
   b. Outlaw
   c. Charlatan
   d. Delinquent

39. Which of the following is a logical conclusion based on the information that is provided within the passage?
   a. Like Elizabeth I, Charles II never married and thus never had children.
   b. The English people were relieved each time that James II's wife Mary lost another child, as this prevented the chance of a Catholic monarch.
   c. Charles I's beheading had less to do with religion than with other political problems that England was facing.
   d. Unlike his son and grandsons, King James I had no Catholic leanings and was a faithful follower of the Protestant Church of England.

40. Based on the information that is provided within the passage, which of the following can be inferred about King James II's son?
   a. Considering his resemblance to King James II, the young James was very likely the legitimate child of the king and the queen.
   b. Given the queen's previous inability to produce a healthy child, the English and the Lowland Scots were right in suspecting the legitimacy of the prince.
   c. James "the Pretender" was not as popular among the Highland clans as his son Bonnie Prince Charlie.
   d. James was unable to acquire the resources needed to build the army and plan the invasion that his son succeeded in doing.

41. The use of the word *ostensibly* in the final paragraph suggests which of the following?
   a. Many of the monarchs of England and Scotland since 1746 have been secretly Catholic.
   b. The Catholic faith is unwelcome in England and Scotland, and Catholics have been persecuted over the centuries.
   c. The Highland clans of Scotland were required to give up their Catholic faith after the Battle of Culloden in 1746.
   d. While Catholics remain within England and Scotland, the two nations profess the Protestant Church of England as the primary church.

42. Which of the following best describes the organization of the information in the passage?
   a. Cause-effect
   b. Chronological sequence
   c. Problem-solution
   d. Comparison-contrast

43. Which of the following best describes the author's intent in the passage?
   a. To persuade
   b. To entertain
   c. To express feeling
   d. To inform

Questions 44 – 46 pertain to the following passage:
   The instructor of a history class has just finished grading the essay exams from his students, and the results are not good. The essay exam was worth 70% of the final course score. The highest score in the class was a low B, and more than half of the class of 65 students failed the exam. In view of this, the instructor reconsiders his grading plan for the semester and sends out an email message to all students.

Dear Students:

The scores for the essay exam have been posted in the online course grade book. By now, many of you have probably seen your grade and are a little concerned. (And if you're not concerned, you should be--at least a bit!) At the beginning of the semester, I informed the class that I have a strict grading policy and that all scores will stand unquestioned. With each class comes a new challenge, however, and as any good instructor will tell you, sometimes the original plan has to change. As a result, I propose the following options for students to make up their score:

1) I will present the class with an extra credit project at the next course meeting. The extra credit project will be worth 150% of the point value of the essay exam that has just been completed. While I will not drop the essay exam score, I will give you more than enough of a chance to make up the difference and raise your overall score.

2) I will allow each student to develop his or her own extra credit project. This project may reflect the tenor of option number 1 (above) but will allow the student to create a project more in his or her own line of interest. Bear in mind, however, that this is more of a risk. The scoring for option number 2 will be more subjective to whether or not I feel that the project is a successful alternative to the essay exam. If it is, the student will be awarded up to 150% of the point value of the essay exam.

3) I will provide the class with the option of developing a group project. Students may form groups of 3 to 4 and put together an extra credit project that reflects a stronger response to the questions in the essay exam. This extra credit project will also be worth 150% of the point value of the essay exam. Note that each student will receive an equal score for the project, so there is a risk in this as well. If you are part of a group in which you do most of the work, each member of the group will receive equal credit for it. The purpose of the group project is to allow students to work together and arrive at a stronger response than if each worked individually.

If you are interested in pursuing extra credit to make up for the essay exam, please choose <u>one</u> of the options above. No other extra credit opportunities will be provided for the course.

Good luck!

Dr. Edwards

44. Which of the following describes this type of writing?
   a. Technical
   b. Narrative
   c. Persuasive
   d. Expository

45. Which of the following best describes the instructor's purpose in writing this email to his students?
   a. To berate students for the poor scores that they made on the recent essay exam.
   b. To encourage students to continue working hard in spite of failure.
   c. To give students the opportunity to make up the bad score and avoid failing the course.
   d. To admit that the essay exam was likely too difficult for most students.

46. Which of the following offers the best summary for the instructor's motive in sending the email to the students?
A) By now, many of you have probably seen your grade and are a little concerned. (And if you're not concerned, you should be--at least a bit!)
B) With each class comes a new challenge, however, and as any good instructor will tell you, sometimes the original plan has to change.
C) The purpose of the group project is to allow students to work together and arrive at a stronger response than if each worked individually.
D) At the beginning of the semester, I informed the class that I have a strict grading policy and that all scores will stand unquestioned.

Questions 47 & 48 pertain to the following passage:
The following memo was posted to a company message board for all employees to review.

To all employees:

It has come to my attention that food items are disappearing from the refrigerator in the break room. Despite the fact that many of the items are unlabeled, they still belong to the individuals who brought them. Because of the food thefts, a number of employees have gone without lunch or have had to purchase a lunch after already bringing one for the day. This is both inconvenient and costly.

This is also unacceptable. Our company prides itself on hiring employees who respect others, and there is no excuse for taking what does not belong to you. Any employee caught taking an item out of the refrigerator that does not belong to him or her risks termination. (As a quick reminder, we encourage those who bring food items to label those items.) Demonstrate courtesy to your colleagues, and respect what is theirs.

In other words, if you didn't bring it, don't eat it.

Alicia Jones

Human Resources Manager

47. Which of the following is the human resources manager's intent in the memo?
   a. To persuade
   b. To entertain
   c. To inform
   d. To express feelings

48. Which of the following explains the reason for the parenthetical note about employees labeling their food items?
    a. The labeling represents a kind of courtesy to the other employees to show which items belong to whom.
    b. The labeling ensures that the company will know whether or not an employee is removing his or her own item.
    c. The labeling represents a rule for employees who bring food, and the company can terminate employees that do not label food items.
    d. The labeling will enable the company to keep track of what is in the refrigerator and ensure that all employees are eating lunch.

Mathematics Test

DIRECTIONS: The mathematics practice test you are about to take is multiple-choice with only one correct answer per question. Read each test item and circle your answer on the answer sheet below. When you have completed the practice test, you may check your answers with those on the answer key that follows the test.

Answer Sheet

1.	a	b	c	d		18.	a	b	c	d
2.	a	b	c	d		19.	a	b	c	d
3.	a	b	c	d		20.	a	b	c	d
4.	a	b	c	d		21.	a	b	c	d
5.	a	b	c	d		22.	a	b	c	d
6.	a	b	c	d		23.	a	b	c	d
7.	a	b	c	d		24.	a	b	c	d
8.	a	b	c	d		25.	a	b	c	d
9.	a	b	c	d		26.	a	b	c	d
10.	a	b	c	d		27.	a	b	c	d
11.	a	b	c	d		28.	a	b	c	d
12.	a	b	c	d		29.	a	b	c	d
13.	a	b	c	d		30.	a	b	c	d
14.	a	b	c	d		31.	a	b	c	d
15.	a	b	c	d		32.	a	b	c	d
16.	a	b	c	d		33.	a	b	c	d
17.	a	b	c	d		34.	a	b	c	d

1. Which of the following is the percent equivalent of 0.0016?
   a. 16%
   b. 160%
   c. 1.6%
   d. 0.16%

2. Curtis is taking a road trip through Germany, where all distance signs are in metric. He passes a sign that states the city of Dusseldorf is 45 kilometers away. Approximately how far is this in miles?
   a. 42 miles
   b. 37 miles
   c. 28 miles
   d. 16 miles

3. Which of the following is the Roman numeral representation for the year 1768?
   a. MDCCLXVIII
   b. MMCXLVIII
   c. MDCCCXLV
   d. MDCCXLIII

4. It is 18 degrees Celsius at Essie's hotel in London. What is the approximate temperature in degrees Fahrenheit?
   a. 25
   b. 48
   c. 55
   d. 64

5. Pernell's last five consecutive scores on her chemistry exams were as follows: 81, 92, 87, 89, 94. What is the approximate average of her scores?
   a. 81
   b. 84
   c. 89
   d. 91

6. What is the *median* of Pernell's scores, as listed in the question above?
   a. 87
   b. 89
   c. 92
   d. 94

7. Gordon purchased a television when his local electronics store had a sale. The television was offered at 30% off its original price of $472. What was the sale price that Gordon paid?
   a. $141.60
   b. $225.70
   c. $305.30
   d. $330.40

8. $\frac{2}{3} \div \frac{4}{15} \times \frac{5}{8}$

Simplify the expression above. Which of the following is correct?

    a. $1\frac{9}{16}$

    b. $1\frac{1}{4}$

    c. $2\frac{1}{8}$

    d. 2

9. 0.0178 x 2.401

Simplify the expression above. Which of the following is correct?

    a. 2.0358414

    b. 0.0427378

    c. 0.2341695

    d. 0.3483240

10. Murray makes $1143.50 for each pay period, and the payments are deposited into his checking account twice a month. His monthly expenses currently include rent at $900 per month, utilities at $250 per month, car insurance at $45 per month, and the cost of food at $300 per month. Murray is trying to put away some money into a separate savings account each month, but he also wants to make sure he has at least $300 left over from his monthly expenses before putting any money into savings. Calculating all of Murray's monthly expenses, including the $300 he wants to keep in his checking account, how much money can he put into the savings account each month?

    a. $192

    b. $292

    c. $392

    d. $492

11. $4(2x - 6) = 10x - 6$

Solve for x above. Which of the following is correct?

    a. 5

    b. -7

    c. -9

    d. 10

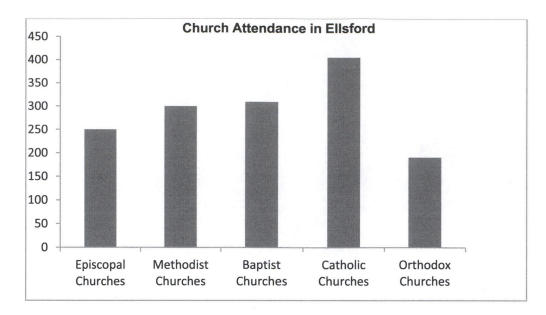

Church Attendance in Ellsford

12. The graph above shows the weekly church attendance among residents in the town of Ellsford, with the town having five different denominations: Episcopal, Methodist, Baptist, Catholic, and Orthodox. Approximately what percentage of church-goers in Ellsford attends Catholic churches?
    a. 23%
    b. 28%
    c. 36%
    d. 42%

13. Erma has her eye on two sweaters at her favorite clothing store, but she has been waiting for the store to offer a sale. This week, the store advertises that all clothing purchases, including sweaters, come with an incentive: 25% off a second item of equal or lesser value. One sweater is $50 and the other is $44. If Erma purchases the sweaters during the sale, what will she spend?
    a. $79
    b. $81
    c. $83
    d. $85

14. Sara plans to set up a booth at an industry fair. The cost for the booth is $500. Additionally, she is planning to give each person who visits the booth a pamphlet about her company and a key chain with the company's logo on it. Fair attendance is expected to be around 1500 people, but Sara expects that she will have only half that many people stop by the booth. As a result, she is only planning to bring pamphlets and key chains for 750 people. The cost of each pamphlet is $0.25 and the cost for each key chain is $0.75. What will Sara's overall cost be?
    a. $750
    b. $900
    c. $1000
    d. $1250

15. $4\frac{2}{3} \div 1\frac{1}{6}$

Simplify the expression above. Which of the following is correct?

  a. 2

  b. $3\frac{1}{3}$

  c. 4

  d. $4\frac{1}{2}$

16. 1.034 + 0.275 – 1.294

Simplify the expression above. Which of the following is correct?

  a. 0.015

  b. 0.15

  c. 1.5

  d. -0.15

17. $(2x + 4)(x – 6)$

Simplify the expression above. Which of the following is correct?

  a. $2x^2 + 8x – 24$

  b. $2x^2 + 8x + 24$

  c. $2x^2 – 8x + 24$

  d. $2x^2 – 8x – 24$

18. On the back of a video case, Digby notices that the listed date of production is MCMXCIV. What is this date in Arabic numerals?

  a. 1991

  b. 1994

  c. 1987

  d. 2003

19. If Stella's current weight is 56 kilograms, which of the following is her approximate weight in pounds. (Note: 1 kilogram is approximately equal to 2.2 pounds.)

  a. 123 pounds

  b. 110 pounds

  c. 156 pounds

  d. 137 pounds

20. Zander is paid $8.50 per hour at his full-time job. He typically works there from 8 AM to 5 PM each weekday, with a one-hour lunch break. The job offers no vacation benefits, so if Zander does not work, he does not get paid. Last week, he worked his full daily schedule of 8 hours each day, except for Wednesday when he left at 3:30 PM. Zander did take his lunch break that day. Which of the following is Zander's pay for the week?

  a. $318.50

  b. $327.25

  c. $335.75

  d. $340

21. $|2x - 7| = 3$
Solve the expression above for x. Which of the following is correct?
    a. $x = 4, 1$
    b. $x = 3, 0$
    c. $x = -2, 6$
    d. $x = 5, 2$

22. Between the years 2000 and 2010, the number of births in the town of Daneville increased from 1432 to 2219. Which of the following is the approximate percent of increase in the number of births during those ten years?
    a. 55%
    b. 36%
    c. 64%
    d. 42%

23. $\frac{1}{4} \times \frac{3}{5} \div 1\frac{1}{8}$
Simplify the expression above. Which of the following is correct?
    a. $\frac{8}{15}$
    b. $\frac{27}{160}$
    c. $\frac{2}{15}$
    d. $\frac{27}{40}$

24. While at the local ice skating rink, Cora went around the rink 27 times total. Cora slipped and fell 20 of the 27 times she skated around the rink. What approximate percentage of the times around the rink did Cora *not* slip and fall?
    a. 37%
    b. 74%
    c. 26%
    d. 15%

25. For her science project, Justine wants to develop a chart that shows the average monthly rainfall in her town. Which type of chart or graph is most appropriate?
    a. Circle graph
    b. Bar graph
    c. Pie chart
    d. Line graph

26. $3\frac{1}{6} - 1\frac{5}{6}$
Simplify the expression above. Which of the following is correct?
    a. $2\frac{1}{3}$
    b. $1\frac{1}{3}$
    c. $2\frac{1}{9}$
    d. $\frac{5}{6}$

27. Four more than a number, x, is 2 less than $\frac{1}{3}$ of another number, y.
Which of the following algebraic equations correctly represents the sentence above?

    a. $x + 4 = \frac{1}{3}y - 2$

    b. $4x = 2 - \frac{1}{3}y$

    c. $4 - x = 2 + \frac{1}{3}y$

    d. $x + 4 = 2 - \frac{1}{3}y$

28. $\dfrac{2xy^2 + 16x^2y - 20xy + 8}{4xy}$

Which of the following expressions is equivalent to the one listed above?

    a. $\frac{2}{y} + 4x - 2xy + 2$

    b. $2y + x^2y - 5 + \frac{xy}{2}$

    c. $\frac{y}{2} + 4x - 5 + \frac{2}{xy}$

    d. $\frac{x}{2} + 4xy - 16 + 2$

29. $4x - 6 \geq 2x + 4$
Solve the inequality above for x. Which of the following is correct?

    a. $x \geq 5$

    b. $x \geq 8$

    c. $x \leq 2$

    d. $x \geq 0$

Question 30 pertains to the following graph:

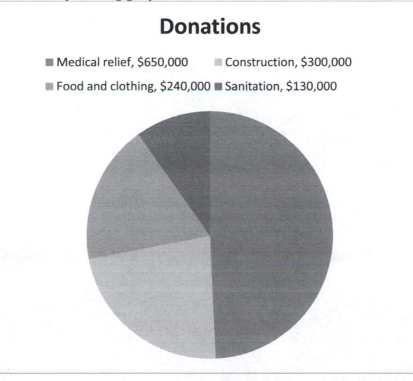

30. After a hurricane struck a Pacific island, donations began flooding into a disaster relief organization. The organization provided the opportunity for donors to specify where they wanted the money to be used, and the organization provided five options. When the organization tallied the funds received, they allotted each to the designated need. Reviewing the chart above, what percentage of the funds was donated to support construction costs?

 a. 49%
 b. 23%
 c. 18%
 d. 10%

31. Margery is planning a vacation, and she has added up the cost. Her round-trip airfare will cost $572. Her hotel cost is $89 per night, and she will be staying at the hotel for five nights. She has allotted a total of $150 for sightseeing during her trip, and she expects to spend about $250 on meals. As she books the hotel, she is told that she will receive a discount of 10% per night off the price of $89 after the first night she stays there. Taking this discount into consideration, what is the amount that Margery expects to spend on her vacation?

 a. $1328.35
 b. $1373.50
 c. $1381.40
 d. $1417.60

32. $\dfrac{7}{3}, \dfrac{9}{2}, \dfrac{10}{9}, \dfrac{7}{8}$

Arrange the numbers above from least to greatest. Which of the following is correct?

 a. $\dfrac{10}{9}, \dfrac{7}{3}, \dfrac{9}{2}, \dfrac{7}{8}$
 b. $\dfrac{9}{2}, \dfrac{7}{3}, \dfrac{10}{9}, \dfrac{7}{8}$
 c. $\dfrac{7}{3}, \dfrac{9}{2}, \dfrac{10}{9}, \dfrac{7}{8}$
 d. $\dfrac{7}{8}, \dfrac{10}{9}, \dfrac{7}{3}, \dfrac{9}{2}$

33. Which of the following is the closest approximation of $\sqrt{30}$?

 a. 5.8
 b. 5.6
 c. 5.5
 d. 5.3

34. $7 + 4^2 - (5 + 6 \times 3) - 10 \times 2$
Simplify the expression above. Which of the following is correct?

 a. -23
 b. -20
 c. 23
 d. 20

Science Test

DIRECTIONS: The science and technical reasoning practice test you are about to take is multiple-choice with only one correct answer per question. Read each test item and circle your answer on the answer sheet below. When you have completed the practice test, you may check your answers with those on the answer key that follows the test.

Answer Sheet

1.	a	b	c	d		28.	a	b	c	d
2.	a	b	c	d		29.	a	b	c	d
3.	a	b	c	d		30.	a	b	c	d
4.	a	b	c	d		31.	a	b	c	d
5.	a	b	c	d		32.	a	b	c	d
6.	a	b	c	d		33.	a	b	c	d
7.	a	b	c	d		34.	a	b	c	d
8.	a	b	c	d		35.	a	b	c	d
9.	a	b	c	d		36.	a	b	c	d
10.	a	b	c	d		37.	a	b	c	d
11.	a	b	c	d		38.	a	b	c	d
12.	a	b	c	d		39.	a	b	c	d
13.	a	b	c	d		40.	a	b	c	d
14.	a	b	c	d		41.	a	b	c	d
15.	a	b	c	d		42.	a	b	c	d
16.	a	b	c	d		43.	a	b	c	d
17.	a	b	c	d		44.	a	b	c	d
18.	a	b	c	d		45.	a	b	c	d
19.	a	b	c	d		46.	a	b	c	d
20.	a	b	c	d		47.	a	b	c	d
21.	a	b	c	d		48.	a	b	c	d
22.	a	b	c	d		49.	a	b	c	d
23.	a	b	c	d		50.	a	b	c	d
24.	a	b	c	d		51.	a	b	c	d
25.	a	b	c	d		52.	a	b	c	d
26.	a	b	c	d		53.	a	b	c	d
27.	a	b	c	d		54.	a	b	c	d

1. The first four steps of the scientific method are as follows:
    I. Identify the problem
    II. Ask questions
    III. Develop a hypothesis
    IV. Collect data and experiment on that data
Which of the following is the next step in the scientific method?
    a. Observe the data
    b. Analyze the results
    c. Measure the data
    d. Develop a conclusion

2. Which of the following best explains the relationship between science and mathematics?
    a. Mathematics offers different levels that science can use, such as geometry and trigonometry.
    b. Science provides the instruments that mathematicians need to complete calculations.
    c. Both help to improve the technology that is required for people to conduct their lives.
    d. Mathematics provides quantitative results that scientists can apply to theories.

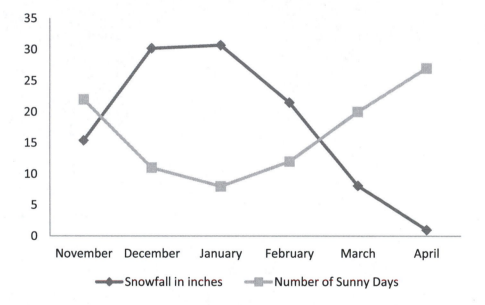

3. The chart above shows the average snowfall in inches for a town on Michigan's Upper Peninsula, during the months November through April. Which of the following can be concluded based on the information that is provided in the chart?
    a. April is not a good month to go skiing in the Upper Peninsula.
    b. Snowfall blocks the sunshine and reduces the number of sunny days.
    c. The fewest sunny days occur in the months with the heaviest snowfall.
    d. There is no connection between the amount of snowfall and the number of sunny days.

4. *Reading long books gives Benezet a headache.*
  War and Peace is a long book.
  Reading War and Peace will give Benezet a headache.
Which of the following correctly describes the conclusion that results from the three statements above?
    a. Inductive
    b. Irrational
    c. Relativistic
    d. Deductive

5. Every time Adelaide visits Ireland, it rains in Dublin. So far, Adelaide has visited Ireland seventeen times in the last three years, and she will visit Ireland again next week.
Which of the following is an *inductive* conclusion to the statements above?
    a. Adelaide should avoid Dublin during her visit.
    b. Adelaide should expect rain in Dublin next week.
    c. Adelaide's visits coincide with the rainy season in Ireland.
    d. Adelaide should put off her trip for a week to avoid the rain.

6. The two criteria for classifying epithelial tissue are *cell layers* and _____.
Which of the following completes the sentence above?
    a. Cell composition
    b. Cell absorption
    c. Cell shape
    d. Cell stratification

7. Which of the following types of connective tissue does *not* have its own (and thus limited) blood supply?
    a. Ligaments
    b. Adipose
    c. Bone
    d. Cartilage

8. Which of the following describes the number of organ systems that are in the human body?
    a. 12
    b. 15
    c. 9
    d. 11

9. Which element within the respiratory system is responsible for removing foreign matter from the lungs?
    a. Bronchial tubes
    b. Cilia
    c. Trachea
    d. Alveoli

10. Organized from high to low, the hierarchy of the human body's structure is as follows: organism, organ systems, organs, tissues. Which of the following comes next?
   a. Molecules
   b. Atoms
   c. Cells
   d. Muscle

Questions 11-16 pertain to the following chart:

Periodic Table

1 IA																	18 VIIIA
1 H 1.01	2 IIA											13 IIIA	14 IVA	15 VA	16 VIA	17 VIIA	**2 He** 4.00
3 Li 6.94	**4 Be** 9.01											**5 B** 10.81	**6 C** 12.01	**7 N** 14.01	**8 O** 16.00	**9 F** 19.00	**10 Ne** 20.18
11 Na 22.99	**12 Mg** 24.31	3 IIIB	4 IVB	5 VB	6 VIB	7 VIIB	8	9 VIIIB	10	11 IB	12 IIB	**13 Al** 26.98	**14 Si** 28.09	**15 P** 30.97	**16 S** 32.07	**17 Cl** 35.45	**18 Ar** 39.95
19 K 39.1	**20 Ca** 40.08	**21 Sc** 44.96	**22 Ti** 47.88	**23 V** 50.94	**24 Cr** 52.00	**25 Mn** 54.94	**26 Fe** 55.85	**27 Co** 58.93	**28 Ni** 58.69	**29 Cu** 63.55	**30 Zn** 65.39	**31 Ga** 69.72	**32 Ge** 72.61	**33 As** 74.92	**34 Se** 78.96	**35 Br** 79.90	**36 Kr** 83.80
37 Rb 85.47	**38 Sr** 87.62	**39 Y** 88.91	**40 Zr** 91.22	**41 Nb** 92.91	**42 Mo** 95.94	**43 Tc** (98)	**44 Ru** 101.07	**45 Rh** 102.91	**46 Pd** 106.42	**47 Ag** 107.87	**48 Cd** 112.41	**49 In** 114.82	**50 Sn** 118.71	**51 Sb** 121.76	**52 Te** 127.6	**53 I** 126.9	**54 Xe** 131.29
55 Cs 132.9	**56 Ba** 137.3	**57 La*** 138.9	**72 Hf** 178.5	**73 Ta** 180.9	**74 W** 183.9	**75 Re** 186.2	**76 Os** 190.2	**77 Ir** 192.2	**78 Pt** 195.1	**79 Au** 197.0	**80 Hg** 200.6	**81 Tl** 204.4	**82 Pb** 207.2	**83 Bi** 209	**84 Po** (209)	**85 At** (210)	**86 Rn** (222)
87 Fr (223)	**88 Ra** (226)	**89 Ac^** (227)	**104 Rf** (261)	**105 Db** (262)	**106 Sg** (263)	**107 Bh** (264)	**108 Hs** (265)	**109 Mt** (268)	**110 Ds** (271)	**111 Rg** (272)							

	58 **Ce** 140.1	59 **Pr** 140.9	60 **Nd** 144.2	61 **Pm** (145)	62 **Sm** 150.4	63 **Eu** 152.0	64 **Gd** 157.3	65 **Tb** 158.9	66 **Dy** 162.5	67 **Ho** 164.9	68 **Er** 167.3	69 **Tm** 168.9	70 **Yb** 173.0	71 **Lu** 175.0
^	90 **Th** 232.0	91 **Pa** (231)	92 **U** 238.0	93 **Np** (237)	94 **Pu** (244)	95 **Am** (243)	96 **Cm** (247)	97 **Bk** (247)	98 **Cf** (251)	99 **Es** (252)	100 **Fm** (257)	101 **Md** (258)	102 **No** (259)	103 **Lr** (260)

*Note: the row labeled with * is the <u>Lanthanide Series</u>, and the row labeled with ^ is the <u>Actinide Series</u>.*

11. On average, how many neutrons does one atom of bromine (Br) have?
   a. 35
   b. 44.90
   c. 45
   d. 79.90

12. On average, how many protons does one atom of zinc (Zn) have?
   a. 30
   b. 35
   c. 35.39
   d. 65.39

13. Which of the following has the highest ionization energy?
    a. Vanadium (V)
    b. Germanium (Ge)
    c. Potassium (K)
    d. Chromium (Cr)

14. Which of the following has the highest electronegativity?
    a. Gallium (Ga)
    b. Thallium (Tl)
    c. Boron (B)
    d. Aluminum (Al)

15. Which of the following would be least likely to chemically bond?
    a. Nitrogen (N)
    b. Sodium (Na)
    c. Calcium (Ca)
    d. Argon (Ar)

16. At 25 °C, there are two elements that exist as liquids: mercury and _____.
    a. Bromine (Br)
    b. Helium (He)
    c. Silicon (Si)
    d. Barium (Ba)

17. Which of the following describes one responsibility of the integumentary system?
    a. Distributing vital substances (such as nutrients) throughout the body
    b. Blocking pathogens that cause disease
    c. Sending leaked fluids from cardiovascular system back to the blood vessels
    d. Storing bodily hormones that influence gender traits

18. When are the *parasympathetic nerves* active within the nervous system?
    a. When an individual experiences a strong emotion, such as fear or excitement
    b. When an individual feels pain or heat
    c. When an individual is either talking or walking
    d. When an individual is either resting or eating

19. Which of the following best describes the relationship between the circulatory system and the integumentary system?
    a. Removal of excess heat from body
    b. Hormonal influence on blood pressure
    c. Regulation of blood's pressure and volume
    d. Development of blood cells within marrow

20. Once blood has been oxygenated, it travels through the pulmonary veins, through the left atrium, and then through the _____ before entering the left ventricle.
    a. Tricuspid valve
    b. Mitral valve
    c. Pulmonary arteries
    d. Aorta

21. *Fungi* are a part of which of the following domains?
    a. Archaea
    b. Archaebacteria
    c. Eubacteria
    d. Eukarya

22. Which of the following are the protein "messengers" that damaged cells release to within the immune system to signal the need for repair?
    a. Cytokines
    b. Perforins
    c. Leukocytes
    d. Interferons

23. The _____ of plant cells are larger than those of eukaryotic cells, because they contain water.
    a. Microtubules
    b. Vacuoles
    c. Flagella
    d. Nuclei

24. The three phases of interphase during mitosis are the following: G_1, G_2, and ____.
    a. V
    b. A
    c. S
    d. R

25. Which of the following is the number of possible *codons* within the code for genetic information?
    a. 16
    b. 32
    c. 64
    d. 128

26. Which of the following can cause mutations in human cells?
    a. Ultraviolet light
    b. Phosphate
    c. Proteins
    d. Nucleotides

27. Fill in the blanks below to complete the equation for photosynthesis:
CO_2 + _____ + Sunlight → _____ + Oxygen
    a. Glucose, Water
    b. Water, Chlorophyll
    c. Water, Glucose
    d. Chlorophyll, Glucose

28. Which of the following describes the purpose of a vaccine?
    a. Repairing damaged tissues that result from virus and/or cancer
    b. Signaling to the body the presence of a disease-causing pathogen
    c. Identifying the disease-causing pathogens that need to be destroyed
    d. Stimulating an infection to allow the body to produce its own antibodies

29. Which of the following cannot exist in RNA?
    a. Uracil
    b. Thymine
    c. Cytosine
    d. Guanine

30. Taking into account the answer the question above, which of the following exists in RNA, place of the substance above?
    a. Thymine
    b. Adenine
    c. Uracil
    d. Cytosine

31. The following four countries are listed in the order of their industrial development, from the greatest to the least amount of industrial development: Japan, Canada, Russia, and Namibia. Which of these countries can be expected to have the highest fertility rates?
    a. Namibia
    b. Canada
    c. Japan
    d. Russia

32. The development of characteristics that allow individuals within a species to survive and reproduce more effectively than others.
Which of the following terms best describes the theory that is defined above?
    a. Mutation
    b. Adaptation
    c. Allele combination
    d. Natural selection

33. In the development of genetic traits, one gene must match to one _____ for the traits to develop correctly.
    a. Codon
    b. Protein
    c. Amino acid
    d. Chromosome

34. Which of the following statements is true about genetic mutations?
    a. Most mutations result from disease.
    b. Mutations are never hereditary.
    c. Mutations due to harmful chemicals are rare.
    d. Most mutations are spontaneous.

35. Positively charged _____ are found *within* the nucleus of an atom, and negatively charged _____ are found *around* the nucleus.
    a. Protons, neutrons
    b. Electrons, neutrons
    c. Protons, electrons
    d. Electrons, protons

36. Which of the following best describes the careful ordering of molecules within solids that have a fixed shape?
    a. Physical bonding
    b. Polar molecules
    c. Metalloid structure
    d. Crystalline order

37. A *weak* bond in DNA often includes a(n) _____ atom.
    a. Oxygen
    b. Nitrogen
    c. Thymine
    d. Hydrogen

38. Which of the following describes the transport network that responsible for the transference of proteins throughout a cell?
    a. Golgi apparatus
    b. Endoplasmic reticulum
    c. Mitochondria
    d. Nucleolus

39. During the *anaphase* of mitosis, the _____, originally in pairs, separate from their daughters and move to the opposite ends (or poles) of the cell.
    a. Chromosomes
    b. Spindle fibers
    c. Centrioles
    d. Nuclear membranes

40. Which of the following is the *shortest* wavelength in the spectrum of electromagnetic waves?
    a. X-ray
    b. Visible
    c. Gamma
    d. Radio

41. The genetic code for DNA is composed of sequences of cytosine, thymine, guanine, and which of the following?
    a. Bromine
    b. Uracil
    c. Nitrogen
    d. Adenine

42. Which of the following offers the best definition of the *Law of Conservation of Energy*?
    a. Energy stores itself for future displacement and in the process preserves itself.
    b. Energy is displaced in motion and replaced in storage.
    c. Energy is never lost but is transferred from one form to another.
    d. Energy causes items in movement to remain thus unless stopped by another force.

43. A(n) _____ is the physical and visible expression of a genetic trait.
    a. Phenotype
    b. Allele
    c. Gamete
    d. Genotype

44. How many protons would a negatively charted isotope of N-12 have?
    a. 5
    b. 7
    c. 10
    d. 12

45. One or more _____ form during a reaction that results in atoms with unbalanced charges.
    a. Protons
    b. Neutrons
    c. Ions
    d. Electrons

46. A substance is considered *acidic* if it has a pH of less than which of the following?
    a. 12
    b. 9
    c. 7
    d. 4

47. Mutations occur as the result of mutagen-induced changes *or* which of the following?
    a. Duplication of a complete genome
    b. Errors during DNA replication
    c. Excision repair inspections of DNA
    d. Presence of germ cells within DNA

48. Which of the following describes the unit that is used to measure the distance between Earth and stars?
    a. Light-years
    b. Parsecs
    c. Nanometers
    d. Angstroms

49. Which of the following would be an example of *potential energy*?
    a. A ballet dancer performing stretches
    b A secretary typing at the computer
    c. A ball being thrown from one person to another
    d. A rubber band stretched to its fullest

50. Which of the following best describes one of the roles of RNA?
   a. Manufacturing the proteins needed for DNA
   b. Creating the bonds between the elements that compose DNA
   c. Sending messages about the correct sequence of proteins in DNA
   d. Forming the identifiable "*double helix*" shape of DNA

51. Which of the following do *catalysts* alter to control the rate of a chemical reaction?
   a. Substrate energy
   b. Activation energy
   c. Inhibitor energy
   d. Promoter energy

52. A metallic ion is considered a(n) _____, while a nonmetallic ion is considered a(n) _____.
   a. Metalloid, anion
   b. Anion, cation
   c. Covalent, cation
   d. Cation, anion

53. An unsaturated hydrocarbon with a double bond is considered a(n) _____, while an unsaturated hydrocarbon with a triple bond is considered a(n) _____.
   a. Alkane, alkyne
   b. Alkyne, alkene
   c. Alkene, alkane
   d. Alkene, alkyne

54. The Punnett square shown here indicates a cross between two parents, one with alleles BB and the other with alleles Bb. Select the correct entry for the upper right box in the Punnett square, which is indicated with the letter, *x*:

	B	B
B		x
b		

   a. Bb
   b. bB
   c. BB
   d. bb

English and Language Usage Test

DIRECTIONS: The English and language usage practice test you are about to take is multiple-choice with only one correct answer per question. Read each test item and circle your answer on the answer sheet below. When you have completed the practice test, you may check your answers with those on the answer key that follows the test.

Answer Sheet

1.	a	b	c	d		23.	a	b	c	d
2.	a	b	c	d		24.	a	b	c	d
3.	a	b	c	d		25.	a	b	c	d
4.	a	b	c	d		26.	a	b	c	d
5.	a	b	c	d		27.	a	b	c	d
6.	a	b	c	d		28.	a	b	c	d
7.	a	b	c	d		29.	a	b	c	d
8.	a	b	c	d		30.	a	b	c	d
9.	a	b	c	d		31.	a	b	c	d
10.	a	b	c	d		32.	a	b	c	d
11.	a	b	c	d		33.	a	b	c	d
12.	a	b	c	d		34.	a	b	c	d
13.	a	b	c	d						
14.	a	b	c	d						
15.	a	b	c	d						
16.	a	b	c	d						
17.	a	b	c	d						
18.	a	b	c	d						
19.	a	b	c	d						
20.	a	b	c	d						
21.	a	b	c	d						
22.	a	b	c	d						

1. Which of the following nouns represents the correct plural form of the word *syllabus*?
a. Syllabus
b. Syllaba
c. Syllabi
d. Syllabis

2. The Welsh kingdom of Gwynedd existed as an independent state from the early 5th century, when the Romans left Britain, until the late 13th century, when the king of England took control of Wales.
Which of the following functions as an adjective in the sentence above?
    a. Independent
    b. Century
    c. Government
    d. Control

3. Hawaii's Big Island, the largest of the eight primary Hawaiian islands, _____ also the youngest of the islands. Which of the following is the correct verb for the subject of the sentence above?
    a. Are
    b. Is
    c. Was
    d. Were

4. Which of the following sentences shows the correct use of quotation marks?
    a. Grady asked Abe, 'Did you know that an earthquake and a tsunami hit Messina, Italy, in 1908?'
    b. Grady asked Abe, "Did you know that an earthquake and a tsunami hit Messina, Italy, in 1908"?
    c. Grady asked Abe, "Did you know that an earthquake and a tsunami hit Messina, Italy, in 1908?"
    d. Grady asked Abe, " 'Did you know that an earthquake and a tsunami hit Messina, Italy, in 1908'?"

5. Cody's dog lost _____ collar, so _____ mom made him rake the leaves to earn the money for a new one. Which of the following sets of words correctly fill in the blanks in the sentence above?
    a. Its; his
    b. It's; his
    c. His; its
    d. His; it's

6. Donald considered the job offer carefully, but he ultimately decided that the low salary was not _____ given his previous experience. Which of the following is the correct completion of the sentence above?
    A) exceptible
    B) acceptible
    C) acepptable
    D) acceptable

7. I'm usually good about keeping track of my keys. I lost them. I spent hours looking for them. I found them in the freezer. Which of the following options best combines the sentences above to show style and clarity?

    a. I lost my keys, even though I'm usually good about keeping track of them. I found them in the freezer and spent hours looking for them.

    b. I spent hours looking for my keys and found them in the freezer. I had lost them, even though I'm usually good about keeping track of them.

    c. I'm usually good about keeping track of my keys, but I lost them. After spending hours looking for them, I found them in the freezer.

    d. I'm usually good about keeping track of my keys, but I lost them in the freezer. I had to spend hours looking for them.

8. It was expected by the administration of Maplewood High School that classes would be canceled because of snow. Which of the following best rewrites the sentences above so that the verbs are active instead of passive?

    a. The administration of Maplewood High School expected to cancel classes because of snow.

    b. The snow caused the administration of Maplewood High School to expect that they would have to cancel classes.

    c. It was expected among the administration of Maplewood High School that the snow would cancel classes.

    d. It was the expectation of the Maplewood High School administration that the snow would cause classes to be canceled.

9. After living in Oak Ridge Missouri all her life, Cornelia was excited about her trip to Prague.
Which of the following best shows the correct punctuation of the city and the state within the sentence above?

    a. After living in Oak Ridge, Missouri, all her life, Cornelia was excited about her trip to Prague.

    b. After living in Oak Ridge, Missouri all her life, Cornelia was excited about her trip to Prague.

    c. After living in Oak, Ridge, Missouri all her life, Cornelia was excited about her trip to Prague.

    d. After living in Oak Ridge Missouri all her life, Cornelia was excited about her trip to Prague.

10. Since each member had a different opinion on the issue, the council decided to rest until _____ could discuss the matter further at a later time. Which of the following pronoun(s) best complete(s) the sentence above?

    a. It

    b. He and she

    c. They

    d. Each

11. The following words all end in the same suffix, *-ism*: polytheism, communism, nationalism. This suffix can apply a variety of meanings to words and suggest a range of possibilities, including a doctrine, a condition, a characteristic, or a state of being. Considering the meaning of these three words, how does the suffix *-ism* apply to all of them?
    a. Doctrine
    b. Condition
    c. Characteristic
    d. State of being

12. Which of the following sentences correctly uses quotes within quotes?
    a. Pastor Bernard read from the book of Genesis: 'And God said, "Let there be light." And there was light.'
    b. Pastor Bernard read from the book of Genesis: "And God said, 'Let there be light.' And there was light."
    c. Pastor Bernard read from the book of Genesis: " 'And God said, Let there be light. And there was light.' "
    d. Pastor Bernard read from the book of Genesis: "And God said, "Let there be light." And there was light."

13. Which of the following is an example of a correctly punctuated sentence?
    a. Beatrice is very intelligent, she just does not apply herself well enough in her classes to make good grades.
    b. Beatrice is very intelligent: she just does not apply herself well enough in her classes to make good grades.
    c. Beatrice is very intelligent she just does not apply herself well enough in her classes to make good grades
    d. Beatrice is very intelligent; she just does not apply herself well enough in her classes to make good grades.

14. Lynton was ready to make a commitment to buying a new car, but he was still unsure about which model would suit him best. Which of the following best removes the nominalization from the sentence above?
    a. Lynton was ready to make a commitment to a new car, but he was still unsure about which model would suit him best.
    b. Lynton was ready to make a commitment to buying a new car, but he was still unsure about the model that would suit him best.
    c. Lynton was ready to commit to buying a new car, but he was still unsure about which model would suit him best.
    d. Lynton was ready to make a commitment to buying a new car, but he was still unsure about which model was best.

15. Which of the following is a compound sentence?
    a. Tabitha and Simon started the day at the zoo and then went to the art museum for the rest of the afternoon.
    b. Tabitha and Simon started the day at the zoo, and then they went to the art museum for the rest of the afternoon.
    c. After starting the day at the zoo, Tabitha and Simon then went to the art museum for the rest of the afternoon.
    d. Tabitha and Simon had a busy day, because they started at the zoo, and then they went to the art museum for the rest of the afternoon.

16. Which of the following follows the rules of capitalization?
    a. Dashiell visited his Cousin Elaine on Tuesday.
    b. Juniper sent a card to her Uncle Archibald who has been unwell.
    c. Flicka and her Mother spent the day setting up the rummage sale.
    d. Lowell and his twin Sister look alike but have very different personalities.

17. Historians tend to count Bede as the Father of English History, because he compiled extensive historical details about early England and wrote the *Ecclesiastical History of the English People.*
Which of the following words does *not* function as a verb in the sentence above?
    a. tend
    b. count
    c. compiled
    d. wrote

18. We cannot allow the budget cuts to _____ the plans to improve education; the futures of _____ children are at stake. Which of the following sets of words correctly fill in the blanks in the sentence above?
    a. effect; your
    b. affect; you're
    c. effect; you're
    d. affect; your

19. The experience of being the survivor of a plane crash left an indelible impression on Johanna, and she suffered from nightmares for years afterwards.
Which of the following best explains the meaning of *indelible* in the sentence above?
    a. candid
    b. permanent
    c. inexpressible
    d. indirect

20. Which of the following sentences contains an incorrect use of capitalization?
    a. For Christmas, we are driving to the South to visit my grandmother in Mississippi.
    b. Last year, we went to East Texas to go camping in Piney Woods.
    c. Next month, we will visit my Aunt Darla who lives just East of us.
    d. When my sister-in-law Susan has her baby, I will take the train north to see her.

21. Which of the following nouns is in the correct plural form?
    a. phenomena
    b. mother-in-laws
    c. deers
    d. rooves

22. Which of the following sentences is grammatically correct?
    a. Krista was not sure who to hold responsible for the broken window.
    b. Krista was not sure whom was responsible for the broken window.
    c. Krista was not sure whom to hold responsible for the broken window.
    d. Krista was not sure on who she should place responsibility for the broken window.

23. Irish politician Constance Markiewicz was the first woman elected to the British House of Commons, but she never served in that capacity due to her activity in forming the Irish Republic.

The word *capacity* functions as which of the following parts of speech in the sentence above?

    a. Verb
    b. Noun
    c. Adverb
    d. Pronoun

24. Which of the following sentences represents the best style and clarity of expression?

    a. Without adequate preparation, the test was likely to be a failure for Zara
    b. The test was likely to be a failure for Zara without adequate preparation
    c. Without adequate preparation, Zara expected to fail the test
    d. Zara expected to fail the test without adequate preparation

25. Valerie refused to buy the television, because she claimed that the price was exorbitant and _____. Which of the following phrases best completes the meaning of the sentence in the context of the word *exorbitant*?

    a. the quality too low for the cost
    b. within the expected price range of similar televisions
    c. much better than she had expected it to be
    d. far exceeding the cost of similar televisions

26. Which of the following sentences contains a correct example of subject-verb agreement?

    a. All of the board members are in agreement on the issue.
    b. Each of the students were concerned about the test scores for the final exam.
    c. Neither of the children are at home right now.
    d. Any of the brownie recipes are perfect for the bake sale.

27. Clemence and I went to the library together, and then _____ stopped to get some coffee.

Which of the following phrases correctly fills in the blanks in the sentence above?

    a. her and I
    b. her and me
    c. she and I
    d. me and her

28. Burton sent the Christmas card to ____ and ____. Which of the following sets of words correctly fills in the blanks in the sentence above?

    a. her; me
    b. she; me
    c. her; I
    d. she; I

29. Which of the following is a simple sentence?

    a. Phillippa walked the dog, and Primula gave the dog a bath.
    b. Phillippa walked and bathed the dog, and Primula helped.
    c. Phillippa walked the dog, while Primula gave the dog a bath.
    d. Phillippa and Primula walked the dog and gave the dog a bath.

30. After the natural disaster struck the county of Hillsborough in Florida, the president declared a state of emergency for that region and promised immediate aid. Which of the following words or phrases in the sentence above should be capitalized?
    a. county
    b. president
    c. state of emergency
    d. aid

31. After his first three-act drama received great critical acclaim, Erastus is on his way to becoming a respected and established _____ in the community. Which of the following correctly completes the sentence above?
    a. play wright
    b. play write
    c. playwright
    d. play-write

32. Which of the following sentences is most correct in terms of style, clarity, and punctuation?
    a. The possible side effects of the medication that the doctor had prescribed for her was a concern for Lucinda, and she continued to take the medication.
    b. The medication that the doctor prescribed had side effects concerning Lucinda who continued to take it.
    c. Lucinda was concerned about side effects from the medication that her doctor had prescribed, so she continued to take it.
    d. Although Lucinda was concerned about the possible side effects, she continued to take the medication that her doctor had prescribed for her.

33. The jury reentered the courtroom after reaching ____ decision. Which of the following correctly completes the sentence above?
    a. it's
    b. they're
    c. its
    d. their

34. Amber was quick to _____ Romy on the way that she had arranged the eclectic pieces of furniture to _____ one another.
Which of the following sets of words correctly fills in the blanks in the sentence above?
    a. compliment; complement
    b. compliment; compliment
    c. complement; compliment
    d. complement; complement

Answer Explanations

Reading Answer Explanations

1. C: To *assuage* is to lessen the effects of something, in this case Adelaide's guilt over eating the piece of cheesecake. The context of the sentence also suggests that she feels sorry for eating it and wants to compensate the following day.

2. A: If Hilaire's vocabulary needs a boost, he needs a thesaurus, which provides a range of synonyms (or antonyms) for words. A dictionary is useful for word meanings, but it will not necessarily assist Hilaire in improving the words he already has in his papers. A Latin dictionary makes little sense in this case, since Hilaire needs to find stronger words in English instead of studying word origins or applying a translation. The encyclopedia is also irrelevant, particularly since the professor already approves of Hilaire's work and is not asking him to research further.

3. A: To find information on Freud's psychological theories, Lise should go to class 100.

4. C: In this case, Lise needs to find a work of literature instead of a work of psychology, so she should consult the 800s.

5. B: To study Jewish traditions further, Lise should consult the 200s, which is devoted to books on religion.

6. D: The first century comprises the years leading up to 100 AD. That means that all first century emperors will have reigns before 100 AD. Hadrian's reign began in 117 AD, so he belongs in the second century instead of the first.

7. A: The sentence indicates a contrast between the appearance and the reality. Enzo's friends believe him to be wealthy, due to the large home that he inherited, but he is actually penniless.

8. B: The word SORT results from following all of the directions that are provided.

9. B: The enrollment in 2001 falls directly between 2000 and 2500, so 2300 is accurate. Note that the enrollment for 2000 falls much closer to 2000, so 2100 is a best estimate for that year.

10. C: The tuition appears to rise alongside the enrollment, until the year 2009 when it jumps significantly. Since the enrollment between 2008 and 2009 does not justify the immediate jump in income for the school, an increase in tuition costs makes sense.

11. C: The word "sic" is Latin for "as such" or "so." It is used to indicate an error on the part of the original author and is used most often when writers are quoting someone else. If the journalist includes the letter as written by the defendant, this is a natural way to show that the misspelling of "guilty" is the responsibility of the defendant and not a typographical error on the part of the journalist.

12. C: The passage is *expository* in the sense that it looks more closely into the mysteries of the Bermuda Triangle and *exposes* information about what researchers have studied and now believe.

13. D: This sentence is the best summary statement for the entire passage, because it wraps up clearly what the author is saying about the results of studies on the Bermuda Triangle.

14. A: Of all the sentences provided, this is the most likely one with which the author would agree. The passage suggests that most of the "mysteries" of the Bermuda Triangle can be explained in a reasonable way. The passage mentions that some expand the Triangle to the Azores, but this is a point of fact, and the author makes no mention of whether or not this is in error. The author quotes the Navy's response to the disappearance of the planes, but there is no reason to believe the author questions this response. The author raises questions about the many myths surrounding the Triangle, but at no point does the author connect these myths with what are described as accidents that fall "within the expected margin of error."

15. C: The inclusion of the statement about the ships from East Asia is an opinion statement, as the author provides no support or explanation. The other statements within the answer choices offer supporting evidence and explanatory material, making them acceptable for an expository composition.

16. A: In this case, the italics suggest a conversation or a dialogue that is occurring between Judith and Martin. While quotation marks are standard for dialogue, the use of italics here is consistent in representing the conversation effectively.

17. B: Only the word *introspection* can fall between *intrauterine* and *invest*. The words *intransigent* and *intone* come before, and the word *investiture* follows.

18. D: The context of the sentence suggests a positive response from the public, so the word *glorify* makes sense as a definition here. There is nothing about the public's response that suggests they criticize or betray him, and the actor's management working to keep information about him private would indicate that the public is not given the opportunity to sympathize with him.

19. D: The spaghetti and the garlic bread are definitely concerns for Ninette if she is unable to consume products with wheat in them. With all other meals, there appear to be gluten-free options that she can eat.

20. C: A discussion of Shakespeare's dramatic works has no place in a chapter that describes his life before he was famous. All other options make sense in a chapter about his formative years and his experiences prior to moving to London and achieving fame.

21. A: The indented portion of the passage indicates that the writer of the letter to the editor is quoting another source (identified as an article by Dr. James Duncan). For long quotes (longer than three lines), it is standard to indent. Shorter quotes (those shorter than three lines) are typically placed in quotation marks and included within the main text of the paragraph.

22. B: The context of the passage suggests that the defense attorney successfully *cleared* his client. To *dismiss* his client would make little sense here. To *condemn* his client would go against his job description, and to *forgive* is not his job–that is the job of the state after the jury reaches its decision.

23. B: This question and the two that follow require simple multiplication and addition. The school needs 500 of each type of textbook. Textbook Central's price for the entire transaction is $47,750 ($4350 and $5200 for each group of 100 textbooks that are purchased). The only textbook supplier with the potential for a competitive price is Textbook Mania, but that company's total price is $48,250. Bookstore Supply's total cost is $48,375. University Textbook's total cost is $48,000.

24. B: Once again, Textbook Central prevails. In this case, it is not even necessary to do the calculations. The cost for composition textbooks is $4350 (per 100) and for linguistics textbooks is $6550 (per 100). The lower cost for the composition textbooks–$150 less per 100 than the closest company in cost–outweighs the slight difference in cost for the linguistics textbooks.

25. C: This question does not require any math. Bookstore Supply has the lowest cost of the four for the technical writing textbooks, and it has a comparable cost to University Textbook for the world literature textbooks. The slight difference for the technical writing textbooks will make the overall cost lower than University Textbook's and thus give Bookstore Supply the competitive edge in cost.

26. D: The key words in question 26 are *nautical* and *docked*. This indicates some type of sailing vessel, which is provided in answer choice D.

27. C: It does not require extensive knowledge of geography to know that Oslo, Norway is nowhere near the Mediterranean Sea. Clearly, this city is out of place in the brochure.

28. B: A closer look at the list indicates that the cities are arranged alphabetically by the name of the city. This means that Galveston fits alphabetically between Fort Lauderdale and Miami.

29. D: Answer choice D is the only option that correctly follows the instructions in the question. Sections 4 and 5 are removed; section 1 is placed on the right sides along sections 3 and 2; and there is a circle drawn around the entire shape. Answer choice A places section 1 in the wrong location and fails to switch sections 2 and 5. Answer choice B incorrectly removes section 1 altogether. Answer choice C changes the shape of section 1 to a rectangle and reverses sections 2 and 3.

30. D: Anna is ultimately looking for a good all-around guidebook for the region. *The Top Ten Places to Visit in Brittany* might have some useful information, but it will not provide enough details about hiking trails, beaches, restaurants, and accommodations. *Getting to Know Nantes* limits the information to one city, and Anna's destination in Brittany is not identified. *Hiking Through Bretagne* limits the information to one activity. These three guidebooks might offer great supplemental information, but *The Complete Guide to Brittany* is the most likely to offer *all* of the information that Anna needs for her trip.

31. B: The passage offers details about a process, so it is descriptive in focus. Narrative passages tell a story. Persuasive passages attempt to persuade the reader to believe or

agree with something. Expository passages *expose* an idea, theory, etc. and provide analysis. The passage provided simply tells the reader how to do something.

32. C: Everby Furnace is located under both Furnace Cleaning and Furnace Installation, so that is the best place for Edgar to start in looking for a company to do both tasks.

33. D: Only V&V Furnace Repair mentions 24-hour service and free estimates on the work. Thomas Refrigeration mentions "24-hour emergency service" specifically, but any company that offers 24-hour furnace repair service is offering it to assist clients with emergencies.

34. B: The passage does not state this outright, but the author indicates that the younger sons of King George III began considering the option of marrying and producing heirs *after* Princess Charlotte Augusta died. Since she was the heir-apparent, her death left the succession undetermined. The author mentions very little about any "wrongs" that Victoria's uncles committed, so this cannot be a logical conclusion. The passage says nothing about the Duke of Kent's preference for a male heir over a female. (In fact, it was likely that he was delighted to have any heir.) And the author does not provide enough detail about the relationship between the Duchess of Kent and King William IV to infer logically that his suspicions were "unreasonable" or that the duchess cared only for her daughter's well-being.

35. C: The author actually notes in the last paragraph that Victoria was an "improbable princess who became queen" and the rest of the passage demonstrates how it was a series of small events that changed the course of British succession. The passage is largely factual, so it makes little sense as a persuasive argument. The author mentions the Victorian Era, but the passage is more about Queen Victoria's family background than it is about the era to which she gave her name. And the passage is more about how the events affected Victoria (and through her, England) than it is about the direct effect that George III's sons had on English history.

36. D: This passage is most likely to belong in some kind of biographical reference about Queen Victoria. A scholarly paper would include more analysis instead of just fact. The information in the passage does not fit the genre of mystery at all. And since the passage recounts history, it is not an obvious candidate for a fictional story.

37. D. All other sentences in the passage offer some support or explanation. Only the sentence in answer choice D indicates an unsupported opinion on the part of the author.

38. A: The passage indicates that it was believed the child died and that he was replaced by another child. Since it is unlikely a parent would willingly give up a child, even for such a purpose, the supposed substitution must have been an orphan. The act would have been illegal, but that does not make the child himself an outlaw (answer choice B). An unknowing infant can hardly be accused of being a charlatan (answer choice C), nor is there enough information in the passage to accuse the infant of being a delinquent (answer choice D). It is likely that, if such a fraud was perpetrated, the child was simply an orphan.

39. C: The author actually says, "Charles's own political troubles extended beyond religion in this case, and he was beheaded in 1649." This would indicate that religion was less involved in this situation than in other situations. There is not enough information to infer that Charles II never married; the passage only notes that he had no legitimate children. (In

- 141 -

fact, he had more than ten illegitimate children by his mistresses.) And while the chance of a Catholic king frightened many in England, it is reaching beyond logical inference to assume that people were relieved when the royal children died. Finally, the author does not provide enough detail for the reader to assume that James I had *no* Catholic leanings. The author only says that James recognized the importance of committing to the Church of England.

40. A: The author notes, "In spite of a strong resemblance to the king, the young James was generally rejected among the English and the Lowland Scots, who referred to him as "the Pretender." This indicates that there *was* a resemblance, and this increases the likelihood that the child was, in fact, that of James and Mary Beatrice. Answer choice B is too much of an opinion statement that does not have enough support in the passage. The passage essentially refutes answer choice C by pointing out that James "the Pretender" was welcomed in the Highlands. And there is little in the passage to suggest that James was unable to raise an army and mount an attack.

41. D: The context of the passage would suggest that Catholicism is not necessarily absent in England and Scotland but that the Church of England is accepted as primary. The word *ostensibly* means *evidently* or *on the surface*, but this alone is not enough to suggest that many monarchs have secretly been Catholic. The passage offers no indication that Catholics remain unwelcome; and while persecution against Catholics is a historical fact, the passage offers no discussion about it. Additionally, there is not enough information in the passage to arrive at the conclusion that the Highland clans were required to give up their Catholic faith. It is a possibility, but it cannot be concluded by the use of the word *ostensibly*.

42. B: The passage is composed in a chronological sequence with each king introduced in order of reign.

43. D: The passage is largely informative in focus, and the author provides extensive detail about this period in English and Scottish history. There is little in the passage to suggest persuasion, and the tone of the passage has no indication of a desire to entertain. Additionally, the passage is historical, so the author avoids expressing feelings and instead focuses on factual information (with the exception of the one opinion statement).

44. A: Technical passages focus on presenting specific information and with a tone of formality. Narrative writing focuses on telling a story, and the passage offers no indication of this. Persuasive writing attempts to persuade the reader to agree with a certain position; the instructor offers the students information but leaves the decision up to each student. Expository passages reveal analytical information to the reader. The instructor is more focused on providing the students with information than with offering the students analytical details. (The analysis, it appears, will be up to the students if they choose to complete an extra credit project.)

45. C.: Answer choice C fits the tone of the passage best. The instructor is simply offering students the chance to make up the exam score (which is worth 70% of their grade) and thus avoid failing the course. The instructor does not berate students at any point, nor does the instructor admit that the exam was too difficult. Additionally, the instructor offers encouragement to the students should they choose to complete an extra credit project, but that is not the primary purpose of this email.

46. B: This question asks for the best summary of the instructor's motive. In the opening paragraph, the instructor notes that his original grading plan has to change to reflect the exam scores. Because they were low, he now wants to give students a chance to make up that score. Answer choice B thus summarizes his motive effectively. The instructor introduces his email with the notes about the scores being posted, but, given the information that is provided in the message, this is not the sole motive for his writing. Answer choice A limits the motive to the details about the group project, and the instructor provides three options. Answer choice D overlooks the instructor's further note about how the grading policy sometimes has to bend to reflect circumstances.

47. C: The human resources manager is informing employees about the company's new policy regarding food items in the refrigerator and the consequences for breaking that policy. There is no overt persuasion in the passage–beyond the standard persuasion of telling people the rules and expecting them to follow those rules or face the consequences. (As a persuasive passage focuses on convincing someone to agree with or believe something, persuasion does not apply to this passage.) The memo has no tone of entertainment or the expression of feelings; it is simply informing employees of a new policy.

48. B: There is no mistake in the location of the parenthetical note. It directly follows the statement about possible termination for employees who take food items that do not belong to them. This indicates that the labeling will help the company recognize that employees are removing their own food items from the refrigerator. The human resources manager mentions the importance of respect or courtesy, but this is not the best explanation for the parenthetical note. There is no suggestion of termination for employees that do not label their food; the memo notes only that the company encourages labeling. The memo offers no suggestion that the company is interested in labeling beyond employees being able to eat their own food. There is no reason to believe that the company is trying to ensure that employees actually eat a lunch.

Mathematic Answer Explanations

1. D: To derive a percentage from a decimal, multiply by 100: 0.0016(100) = 0.16%.

2. C: One kilometer is about 0.62 miles, so 45(0.62) is 27.9, or approximately 28 miles.

3. A: In Roman numerals, M is 1000, D is 500, C is 100, L is 50, X is 10, V is 5, and I is 1. For the year 1768, the Roman numeral MDCCLXVIII is correct – representing 1000 + 500 + 200 + 50 + 10 + 5 + 3. MMCXLVIII is 2148 (still yet to be achieved) MDCCCXLV is 1845, and MDCCXLIII is 1743.

4. D: To convert from Celsius to Fahrenheit, start by multiplying by 9 and then dividing by 5. Add 32 to the quotient, and the conversion is complete. For question 4:
$$18(9) = 162$$
$$162/5 = 32.4$$
$$32.4 + 32 = 64.4, \text{ or approximately } 64$$

5. C: To find the average of Pernell's scores, add them up and then divide by the number of scores (5 in this case). In other words,

$$81 + 92 + 87 + 89 + 94 = 443$$
$$443/5 = 88.6, \text{ or approximately } 89$$

6. B: To find the median, list the series of numbers from least to greatest. The middle number represents the median--in this case 81, 87, 89, 92, 94. The number 89 is in the middle, so it is the median.

7. D: The television is 30% off its original price of $472. Therefore, 30% of 472 is 141.60, and 141.60 subtracted from 472 is 330.40. Thus, Gordon pays $330.40 for the television.

8. A: To simplify, proceed in the order of the operations: $\frac{2}{3} \div \frac{4}{15}$ is $\frac{2}{3} \times \frac{15}{4}$, or $\frac{5}{2}$. Next, multiply $\frac{5}{2}$ by $\frac{5}{28}$. The result is $\frac{25}{16}$, or $1\frac{9}{16}$.

9. B: Question 9 is a simple matter of multiplication. The product is 0.0427378.

10. D: Start by multiplying Murray's payment by 2, since he receives this twice a month: $2287. Subtract all of his expenses, including the $300 he plans to keep in his checking account. The amount of $492 is left over, and this is what Murray can plan to put in his savings account each month, as long as his expenses remain the same.

11. C: Multiplying the equation results in the following:

$$8x - 24 = 10x - 6$$
$$-18 = 2x$$
$$x = -\frac{18}{2}, or - 9$$

12. B: Adding up the number of church-goers in Ellsford results in about 1450 residents who attend a church in the town each week. There are approximately 400 people in Ellsford who attend a Catholic church each week. This number represents about 28% of the 1450 church-goers in the town.

13. C: Erma's sale discount will be applied to the less expensive sweater, so she will receive the $44 sweater for 25% off. This amounts to a discount of $11, so the cost of the sweater will be $33. Added to the cost of the $50 sweater, which is not discounted, Erma's total is $83.

14. D: The combined cost of the pamphlets (750 at $0.25 each) and the key chains (750 at $0.75 each) is $750. With the cost of the booth ($500), Erma will pay a total of $1250.

15. C: Turn both expressions into fractions, and then multiply the first by the reverse of the second:

$$\frac{14}{3} \div \frac{7}{6}$$
$$\frac{14}{3} \times \frac{6}{7}$$

The result is the whole number 4.

16. A: Start by adding the first two expressions, and then subtract 1.294 from the sum:

$$1.034 + 0.275 = 1.309$$
$$1.309 - 1.294$$

The result is 0.015.

17. D: Multiply in the required order, and then add: $(2x)(x) + (2x)(-6) + (4)(x) + (4)(-6)$. The result is $2x^2 - 8x - 24$.

18. B: Recall that in Roman numerals, M is 1000, D is 500, C is 100, L is 50, X is 10, V is 5, and I is 1. As a result, the year MCMXCIV is 1994. (Note that the I before the V indicates that the I is subtracted from V: 5 – 1, or 4. In the same way, the C before the M also indicates a subtraction, in this case 100 from 1000, or 900.)

19. A: To find the correct answer, simply multiply 56 by 2.2. The result is 123.2, or approximately 123. This is Stella's weight in pounds.

20. B: To find the correct answer, start by adding up what Zander makes for the four full days he works: $8.50 per hours for 32 hours (four full 8-hour days). The result is $272. Then, add up what Zander makes on Wednesday when he leaves at 3:30 but still takes his standard one-hour lunch break. By leaving at 3:30, Zander only works 6.5 hours that day. At $8.50 per hour, this is $55.25 for the day. Added to $272, the result is $327.25.

21. D: Absolute value is determined by the distance between a number and 0 when plotted on a number line. For instance, the absolute value of –5 is 5. To solve the equation in question 21 for x requires the following:

$$|2x - 7| = 3$$
$$2x - 7 = 3, or\ 2x - 7 = -3$$
$$2x - 7 = 3$$
$$2x = 10, so\ x = 5$$
$$OR$$
$$2x = 4, so\ x = 2$$

The two possible solutions for the absolute value of the equation are 5 and 2.

22. A: Begin by subtracting 1432 from 2219. The result is 787. Then, divide 787 by 1432 to find the percent of increase: 0.549, or 54.9%. Rounded up, this is approximately a 55% increase in births between 2000 and 2010.

23. C: Solve the equation in the order of operations: $\frac{1}{4} \times \frac{3}{5}$, or $\frac{3}{20}$. Follow this up with division, which requires a reversal of the fraction: $\frac{3}{20} \div \frac{9}{8}$, or $\frac{3}{20} \times \frac{8}{9}$. The result is $\frac{2}{15}$.

24. C: Cora did *not* fall 7 out of 27 times. To find the solution, simply divide 7 by 27 to arrive at 0.259, or 25.9%. Rounded up, this is approximately 26%.

25. D: Justine's graph will be charting the amount of rainfall for each month. Line graph indicate change that occurs over a specified period of time, so this is the best type of graph for Justine to use.

26. B: Since the denominator is the same for both fractions, this is simple subtraction. Start by turning each expression into a fraction: $\frac{19}{6} - \frac{11}{6}$. The result is $\frac{8}{6}$, or $1\frac{2}{6} = 1\frac{1}{3}$.

27. A: The expression "Four more than a number, x" can be interpreted as $x + 4$. This is equal to "2 less than $\frac{1}{3}$ of another number, y," or $\frac{1}{3}y - 2$.

28. C: To solve the equation, start by separating each element:
$$\frac{2xy^2 + 16x^2y - 20xy + 8}{4xy}$$
$$\frac{2xy^2}{4xy}, \text{ or } \frac{y}{2}$$
$$\frac{16x^2y}{4xy}, \text{ or } 4x$$
$$-\frac{20xy}{4xy}, \text{ or } -5$$
$$\frac{8}{4xy}, \text{ or } \frac{2}{xy}$$
Combine: $\frac{y}{2} + 4x - 5 + \frac{2}{xy}$.

29. A: To solve, move the terms with x to the same side of the equation and the whole numbers to the other:
$$4x - 6 \geq 2x + 4$$
$$2x \geq 10$$
$$x \geq 5$$
You can test this answer by filling in a number greater than 5 to see if the inequality still holds. For instance with the number 7:
$$4(7) - 6 \geq 2(7) + 4$$
The number 22 (or $28 - 6$) is greater than (though obviously not equal to) 18 (or $14 + 4$), so the inequality works. The only time when the two sides are equal is when $x = 5$.
Note that answer choice B contains a number greater than 5 that also works to make the inequality correct (when the left side of the equation is greater than the right side). The number 8 works only for "greater than," however, and does not solve for "equal to," so answer choice B cannot be the correct answer.

30. B: Start by locating the section of the pie chart that represents construction. It looks close to a quarter of the pie chart, which means that it is probably 23%, but you can verify by adding up the numbers. The total donation amount is about $1.3 million and the amount given for construction is $0.3 million. 0.3/1.3 = 0.23 = 23%.

31. C: Start by adding up the costs of the trip, excluding the hotel cost: $572 + $150 + $250, or $972. Then, calculate what Margery will spend on the hotel. The first of her five nights at the hotel will cost her $89. For each of the other four nights, she will get a discount of 10% per night, or $8.90. This discount of $8.90 multiplied by the four nights is $35.60. The total she would have spent on the five nights without the discount is $445. With the discount, the amount goes down to $409.40. Add this amount to the $972 for a grand total of $1381.40.

32. D: Turn the fractions into mixed numbers to see the amounts more clearly. The result is that $\frac{7}{8}$ is smaller than $\frac{10}{9}$, or $1\frac{1}{9}$, which is smaller than $\frac{7}{3}$, or $2\frac{1}{3}$, which is smaller than $\frac{9}{2}$, or $4\frac{1}{2}$.

33. C: The square root of 25 is 5, and the square root of 36 is 6. The correct answer to the square root of 30 will have to be closely to the mid-point between 5 and 6. As a result, 5.5 is a good place to start testing, and it proves to be correct: $\sqrt{30} = 5.477$. This is approximately 5.5. (In exact terms, 5.5^2 is 30.25, but as this question only asks for the approximation, the answer of 5.5 is correct.) In comparison, 5.3^2 is 28.09; 5.6^2 is 31.36; 5.8^2 is 33.64. None of these is close enough to 30 to be correct.

34. B: Start by calculating the amount in parenthesis, completing the multiplication first: $5 + 6 \times 3$, which is $5 + 18$ or 23. Then calculate the product at the end: 10×2, or 20. Calculate the expression 4^2, for a result of 16, and complete the equation:

$$7 + 16 - 23 - 20$$
$$23 - 23 - 20$$
$$0 - 20, or - 20$$

Science Answer Explanations

1. B: There are six steps in the scientific process, the fifth of which is "Analyze the results" (the results of the experiments that were conducted in step four). The results of step four must be analyzed before reaching the final step, "Develop a conclusion."

2. D: Science and mathematics work together with mathematics offering the quantitative results that scientists can use to apply to their theories and thus prove whether or not they are correct.

3. C: The chart shows two specific changes: snowfall levels from November to April and sunny days from November to April. Based on the chart alone, the only information that can be determined is that the fewest sunny days coincide with the months that have the heaviest snowfall. Anything further reaches beyond the immediate facts of the chart and moves into the territory of requiring other facts. As for answer choice D, it uses the word "relationship," which is not required in the question. The question only asks for what can be concluded.

4. D: Deductive reasoning moves from the general to the specific. In this case, the general statement is that Benezet gets a headache from reading long books. The syllogism moves from the general to the specific by noting that *War and Peace* is a long book, therefore Benezet will likely get a headache from reading it.

5. B: Inductive reasoning moves from the specific to the general. In this case, the specific statement is that there is rain in Dublin every time Adelaide visits Ireland. The syllogism in this case moves from the specific to the general by then noting that Adelaide has visited Ireland 17 times in the last 3 years and that she will visit again next week. This is significant, because it raises the likelihood of rain. There is no guarantee of course, but the question merely asks for the inductive conclusion. To conclude the syllogism inductively, the best answer choice notes that Adelaide should expect rain in Dublin next week. All other answer choices move beyond the immediate syllogism and infer other information. (For instance, the first statement does not note that Adelaide actually visits Dublin but rather that she visits Ireland. It can rain in Dublin without Adelaide being there.) It is also possible to infer

- 147 -

that Adelaide visits Ireland during the rainy season, but that is not a part of the original statement and therefore not possible as an inductive conclusion to the syllogism.

6. C: *Cell layers* and *cell shape* are the criteria for classifying epithelial tissue.

7. A: Ligaments do not have their own blood supply. As a result, ligament injuries tend to take longer to heal because they have a limited blood supply.

8. D: There are 11 organ systems in the human body: circulatory, digestive, endocrine, integumentary, lymphatic, muscular, nervous, reproductive, respiratory, skeletal, and urinary.

9. B: The cilia are the tiny hairs in the respiratory system that are responsible for removing foreign matter from the lungs. The cilia are located within the bronchial tubes, but it is the cilia that have the responsibility for removing inappropriate materials before they enter the lungs.

10. C: Cells come after tissues and are followed by molecules and then atoms at the very bottom of the hierarchy. Muscles are types of tissues, so muscles do not have a separate place in the hierarchy but instead fall within the types of tissues.

11. B: To determine the average number of neutrons in one atom of an element, subtract the atomic mass from the atomic number. For Bromine (Br), subtract its atomic number (35) from its atomic mass (79.9) to acquire the average number of neutrons, 44.9.

12. A: The number of protons is the same as the element's atomic periodic number: in this case, 30 for Zinc (Zn).

13. B: Ionization energy increases across a period (or row), from left to right. In the period containing the four elements listed in question 13, germanium (Ge) is the furthest to the right and thus has the highest ionization energy, also known as ionization potential.

14. C: Electronegativity increases in a group (or column) as the atomic number decreases— or put another way, the lower the atomic number, then the higher the electronegativity. Among the four elements listed in question 14, Boron (B) has the lowest atomic number (5) and thus the highest electronegativity.

15. D: As one of the noble gases, argon (Ar) is neutral and thus has no electrons for chemical bonding. As a result, it as well as the other noble gases in the period can resist chemical bonding.

16. A: Mercury and bromine are the only elements that are recognized as liquids in their natural state.

17. B: The integumentary system includes skin, hair, and mucous, and all are responsible—in part, at least—for blocking disease-causing pathogens from entering the blood stream. The circulatory system distributes vital substances through the body. The lymphatic system sends leaked fluids from the cardiovascular system back to the blood vessels. The reproductive system stores bodily hormones that influence gender traits.

18. D: The *parasympathetic nerves* are active when an individual is either resting or eating. The sympathetic nerves are active when an individual experiences a strong emotion, such as fear or excitement. Feeling pain and heat fall under the responsibility of the sensory neurons. Talking and walking fall under the responsibility of the ganglia within the sensory-somatic nervous system.

19. A: The integumentary system (i.e., the skin, hair, mucous, etc.) coordinates with the circulatory system to remove excess heat from the body. The superficial blood vessels (those nearest the surface of the skin) dilate to allow the heat to exit the body. The hormonal influence on blood pressure is the result of the relationship between the circulatory system and the endocrine system. The urinary system is responsible for assisting in the regulation of blood's pressure and volume. The skeletal system is responsible for assisting in the development of blood vessels within the marrow.

20. B: After the blood has gone through the left atrium, it enters the mitral valve before entering the left ventricle.

21. D: There are three domains: Archaea, Eukarya, and Eubacteria. *Fungi*, along with Plantae, Animalia, and Protista, falls within the Eukarya domain.

22. A: Cytokines signal to cells that damaged tissues need to be repaired. Perforins specifically target viruses and cancers. Leukocytes are the white blood cells that respond when tissues need to be repaired. Interferons help in the response to virus attacks by keeping the virus from replicating and spreading within the body.

23. B: The vacuoles function as a type of storage unit cell needs. In plant cells, the vacuoles are larger than in eukaryotic cells due to the water content that they require for adequate cell pressure.

24. C: The S phase is the third phase of interphase during mitosis.

25. C: The code is composed of the substances within DNA: adenine (A), cytosine (C), guanine (G), and thymine (T). It is possible to make 64 codons from the combination of these letters.

26. A: Ultraviolet light can cause the genetic mutations. Phosphate is a natural part of DNA, as are proteins. In fact, it is the alteration of the natural phosphate structure of the DNA that results in a mutation. Nucleotides also form a natural base within DNA.

27. C: The equation for photosynthesis requires a combination of carbon dioxide (CO_2), water, and sunlight to result in glucose and oxygen.
28. D: The vaccine brings a small amount of an infection into the body to give the body a chance to build up defenses to it by producing antibodies. These antibodies will recognize the disease in the future and prevent contraction of it.

29. B: The substance thymine cannot exist in RNA.

30. C: The substance *uracil* exists in RNA, in place of thymine.

31. A: Scientists have found that fertility rates tend to decrease as societies become more industrialized. As a result, the most industrialized countries typically have low fertility rates, while the least industrialized countries have higher fertility rates. With this in mind, and considering the information provided, Namibia--the least industrialized in the list of nations that is provided--can be expected to have the highest fertility rates.

32. D: Question 32 presents the theory of *natural selection*, or Darwin's theory of the *survival of the fittest*: individuals within a species develop characteristics that allow them to survive and reproduce more effectively (passing on the genes that they carry).

33. B: Each gene must match to a protein for a genetic trait to develop correctly.

34. D: The only true statement among the answer choices is that the majority of mutations are spontaneous. Very few mutations result from disease (although some diseases might result from genetic mutation). Some mutations (such as hemophilia) are indeed hereditary, so they can be passed on through the generations. Harmful chemicals are a known source of genetic mutations, so mutations that result from this source cannot be considered rare.

35. C: Protons are positively charged and found within the nucleus of an atom, while electrons are negatively charged and are found around the nucleus.

36. D: Solids with a fixed shape have a crystalline order that defines and maintains that shape.

37. D: A hydrogen atom creates a weak bond in DNA--in fact, this weak bond is known as a hydrogen bond due to the presence of the hydrogen atom.

38. B: The endoplasmic reticulum is the cell's transport network that moves proteins from one part of the cell to another. The Golgi apparatus assists in the transport but is not the actual transport network. Mitochondria are organelles ("tiny organs") that help in the production of ATP, which the cells need to operate properly. The nucleolus participates in the production of ribosomes that are needed to generate proteins for the cell.

39. A: The chromosomes separate during anaphase and move to the opposite ends of the cells.

40. C: Gamma rays are the shortest wavelengths in the spectrum. From longest to shortest: radio, microwave, infrared, visible, ultraviolet, x-ray, gamma.

41. D: Adenine is the fourth type of nitrogenous base in DNA. Bromine is not part of DNA construction. Uracil is found in RNA but not in DNA.

42. C: The Law of Conservation of Energy states that energy is never actually lost but instead is transferred back and forth from kinetic to potential. Answer choices A and B do not make much sense, and answer choice D reflects Newton's Second Law instead of the Law of Conservation of Energy.

43. A: The physical expression--such as hair color--is the result of the phenotype. The genotype is the basic genetic code.

44. B: Charge and isotope do not affect the number of protons: protons are determined by the atomic number as shown in the periodic table. Nitrogen (N) has an atomic number of 7, so that is the number of protons that a negatively charted isotope of N-12 has.

45. C: An ion results from an imbalance of charges on an atom after a reaction. A neutral atom has an equal number of protons and electrons so the number of positive charges from the protons is balanced by the amount of negative charges from the electrons. When electrons are transferred between atoms during a chemical reaction, an atom will become positively charged if it has lost electrons or negatively charged if it has gained electrons.

46. C: The number of 7 is the "breaking point" between basic and acidic. Above 7 solutions are considered basic; below 7 solutions are considered acidic. For instance, milk, with a pH of 6.5, is actually considered acidic. Bleach, with a pH of 12.5, is considered basic.

47. B: Mutations result from mutagen-induced changes or errors during DNA replication. That being said, DNA replication is a normal activity, so answer choice A cannot be said to cause mutations. Similarly, excision repair (answer choice C) and the presence of germ cells (answer choice D) are normal within DNA, so neither causes mutations. Errors that occur during these processes, however, might.

48. A: Scientists measure the distance between the earth and the stars (including the sun) in light-years, which is calculated as the distance that light will travel in one year.

49. D: Potential energy is energy that *can* be used but is not currently being used. A ballerina doing stretches is using energy. A secretary typing at a computer is also using energy. Note that a great deal of energy does not have to be used for the energy to be considered *kinetic* or in use (as a result of motion). A ball being thrown from one person to another is in motion and thus possesses kinetic energy. A rubber band stretched to its fullest and held, however, is waiting to spring back and possesses *potential* energy, or the energy that is being stored before use.

50. C: RNA has several roles, one of which is to act as the messenger and deliver information about the correct sequence of proteins in DNA. The ribosomes do the actual manufacturing of the proteins. Hydrogen, oxygen, and nitrogen work to create the bonds within DNA. And far from having a double helix shape, RNA has what would be considered a more two-dimensional shape.

51. B: Catalysts alter the activation energy during a chemical reaction and therefore control the rate of the reaction. The substrate is the actual surface that enzymes use during a chemical reaction (and there is no such term as *substrate energy*). Inhibitors and promoters participate in the chemical reaction, but it is the activation energy that catalysts alter to control the overall rate as the reaction occurs.

52. D: A metallic ion is called a *cation*, while a nonmetallic ion is called an *anion*. *Metalloid* refers to a type of element that easily accepts or gives off electrons. The term *covalent* refers to a specific type of bond between elements (that is, when atoms share electrons).
53. D: An *alkene* has a double bond, while an *alkyne* has a triple bond. The *alkane* is the saturated hydrocarbon that is altered to produce the unsaturated hydrocarbons with the double or triple bonds. For instance, ethane is the alkane; ethene is the alkene; ethyne is the alkyne.

54. C: Crossing the corresponding alleles from each parent will yield a result of BB in the upper right box of this Punnett square.

English and Language Usage Answer Explanations

1. C: The word *syllabi* is the correct plural form of *syllabus*. The other answer choices reflect incorrect plural forms. Specifically, *syllabus* does not change the form at all, and the Latin root of *syllabus* would require some change. At the same time, *syllaba*--while an accurate plural for some words with Latin roots--is incorrect in this case. And *syllabis* is a double form of the plural, so it cannot be correct.

2. A: The word *independent* is an adjective that modifies the word *state*, describing the type of state that described the kingdom of Gwynedd. The words *century*, *government*, and *control* are all nouns in this context.

3. B: Correct subject-verb agreement would require the singular verb *is* to accompany the singular subject *Big Island*. Readers should not be distracted by the use of *islands* in the appositive phrase just before the verb. The subject-verb relationship is governed by the word that functions as the subject of the sentence, instead of the noun (or, in some cases, the pronoun) that is closest to the verb.

4. C: Answer choice A is correct, because the quotation is a standard quotation (requiring double quotes) as well as a question. Additionally, the question mark belongs inside the quotation marks. Answer choice A correctly places the question mark inside the quotation marks, but the use of single quotes is incorrect for standard quotations. Answer choice B is incorrect, because it places the question mark outside the quotation marks. Answer choice D uses the layered quotes, which are unnecessary in this case, since the sentence presents only one quotation instead of more than one.

5. A: The word *its* is a possessive pronoun the reflects the collar belonging to the dog, and the use of *his* applies to Cody. Answer choice B incorrectly uses the contraction for *it is*. Answer choice C switches the pronouns so that *its* refers to Cody instead of the dog. Answer choice D does the same thing, except with the contraction for *it is* instead of the possessive pronoun.

6. D: *acceptable* is the correct spelling of the word. All other forms represent incorrect spelling of a commonly misspelled word.

7. C: Answer choice C offers the most effective combination of the sentences with the use of the conjunction *but* and the dependent clause starting with *after*. All other answer choices result in choppy or unclear combinations of the four sentences.

8. A: The original sentence contains two passive usages (*was expected* and *would be canceled*). Neither is necessary; both can be adjusted to improve the clarity of the sentence. Answer choice A best adjusts the passive tense to active. Answer choice B awkwardly makes *snow* the subject of the sentence when *administration* is a more effective subject. Answer choice C simply replaces *by* with *among*, but this does nothing to improve the clarity of the

sentence. Answer choice D offers a nominalization (*expectation*), which clutters the sentence instead of improves it.

9. A: Correct punctuation requires a comma after both city and state when both fall within the sentence, even when the city and state fall within an opening dependent clause that has a comma after it. All answer choices that do not have a comma after the state as well as the city are incorrect. Answer choice C is incorrect because it adds a comma after *Oak* for no clear reason as the name of the city in full is clearly *Oak Ridge*.

10. C: The word *council* is a collective noun that, in this case, represents a group of individuals functioning individually. As a result, *council* is plural, so it needs the plural pronoun *they*. Within the context of the sentence, *he and she* makes no sense, and *each* is singular in this case, so it does not indicate the plural nature of the council.

11. A: The suffix *-ism* here suggests a doctrine that is followed, whether that be the doctrine of polytheism (a religious doctrine), communism (a social doctrine), or nationalism (a political doctrine).

12. B: Question 12 asks for the correct punctuation of layered quotations. Standard American usage requires the double quotes for the first quotation and the single quotes for any quotes within the original quotes. Answer choice B best reflects this with the phrase "Let there be light" representing the quote within the original quotation. Answer choice A reverses the correct usage. Answer choice C incorrectly makes the entire quotation a quote within an otherwise unidentified quote. Answer choice D uses double quotes within the double quotes, which is incorrect in standard American usage.

13. D: The semicolon correctly joins the two sentences. Answer choice A is incorrect, because it uses a comma splice to join two independent clauses. (To join two independent clauses, a comma needs to be accompanied by a coordinating conjunction.) The colon in answer choice B is incorrect because the information in the second clause does not clearly define or explain the previous clause. Answer choice C is incorrect because it offers no punctuation to separate the two independent clauses and thus creates more confusion than clarity.

14. C: Question 14 asks the student to identify and remove the nominalization. In the original sentence, the nominalization is *commitment*. The easiest way to remove the nominalization is to adjust it to the verb *commit*. As a result, answer choice C is the only correct option because it identifies and removes the nominalization.

15. B: Answer choice B contains two independent clauses that are joined with a comma and the coordinating conjunction *and*. Answer choice A, though it contains a compound subject and a compound verb, is still a simple sentence. Answer choice C opens within a dependent clause, so it is a complex sentence. Answer choice D is a compound-complex sentence because it includes a dependent clause as well as two independent clauses.

16. B: Answer choice B correctly capitalizes *Uncle Archibald*, where *Uncle* refers to a specific name. The word *cousin* needs no capitalization, even when it refers to the name of a specific relative. (The only distinctions are when the word is used within a direct address or opens a sentence.) Similarly, *mother* and *sister* do not need to be capitalized unless they are the first word of the sentence or are part of a direct address.

- 153 -

17. B: The word *count* is part of an infinitive phrase (*to count*), and infinitive phrases function as nouns, so the word *count* cannot be a verb. All other answer choices are verbs.

18. D: The word *affect* is a verb in this context and is the correct usage within the sentence. The possessive pronoun *your* also correctly modifies *children*, so answer choice D is correct. All other answer choices incorrectly apply the words to the sentence.

19. B: The context of the sentence suggests that the trauma of surviving the plane crash left long-term memories that haunted Johanna for many years. As a result, *permanent* is the best meaning of *indelible*. The other meanings make little sense in the context of the sentence. The only possible option is *indirect*, but there is nothing about the sentence to suggest that the nightmares are indirect impressions of a traumatic experience.

20. C: The word *east* in answer choice C is simply a directional indication and does not need to be capitalized in the context of the sentence. All other uses of capitalization are correct in the context of the sentences. The word *South* should be capitalized when it refers to a region of the United States (as indicated by the mention of Mississippi). The word *East* should be capitalized when it refers to the region of Texas. And the word *north* does not need to be capitalized when it is simply a directional indication (as in answer choice D).

21. A: The word *phenomena* is the correct plural form of *phenomenon*, so answer choice A is correct. The correct plural form of *mother-in-law* is *mothers-in-law*. The correct plural form of *deer* is just *deer*. The correct plural form of *roof* is *roofs*.

22. C: The word *whom* correctly indicates the objective case--as in "to hold him/her responsible"--so answer choice C is correct. The word *who* in answer choice A incorrectly indicates the subjective case. Similarly, answer choice B is incorrect because the word *who* is the subjective case (instead of the objective case) here. Answer choice D is incorrect because it incorrect applies the objective *whom* instead of the subjective *who*.

23. B: The word *capacity* is a noun in this context, so answer choice B is correct. Because the word functions as the object of the preposition, the options of verb and adverb cannot be correct. Answer choice D is incorrect because the word *capacity* is not a pronoun in any context.

24. C: Answer choice C summarizes the ideas within the sentence simply and clearly. Answer choice A moves the ideas around to make them awkward instead of effective. Answer choice B creates a dangling modifier with the phrase *without adequate protection*, so it cannot be correct. Similarly, answer choice D makes this phrase a dangling modifier that makes the flow of thought awkward instead of clear.

25. D: The context of the sentence suggests that the word *exorbitant* refers to an excessively high cost, so answer choice D is most correct. Answer choice A would be an interesting conclusion to the sentence, but it does not clearly follow the use of *exorbitant*, so it cannot be correct. Answer choices B and C contradict the suggested meaning of *exorbitant*, so both must be incorrect.

26. A: The pronoun *all* is plural, so it requires the plural verb *are*. The pronouns *each* and *neither* are singular and require singular verbs (not provided in answer choices B and C). The pronoun *any* can be either singular or plural depending on the context of the sentence.

In this case, *any* suggests a singular usage, so answer choice D is incorrect with the plural verb.

27. C: The pronouns *she and I* are correctly in the subjective case starting the second independent clause, so answer choice C is correct. All other answer choices contain at least one incorrect objective case usage that cannot function as the subject of the second independent clause.
28. A: Both *her* and *me* are objective case pronouns that accurately function as the object of the preposition *to*. All other answer choices contain at least one incorrect subjective case usage that cannot function as the object of the preposition.

29. D: While answer choice D is arguably the longest of the four sentences, it is actually a simple sentence. It contains a compound subject and a compound verb, but because it represents only one independent clause it still functions as a simple sentence. Answer choices A and B contain two independent clauses and are thus compound sentences. Answer choice C contains a dependent clause, so it is a complex sentence.

30. B: The word *President* should always be capitalized when it refers to the President of the United States, whether or not the President's name is included. All other nouns in this sentence are simple nouns and do not need to be capitalized.

31. C: The word *playwright* is the correct spelling to refer to someone who writes plays. All other forms are incorrect and reflect common confusion about the correct spelling of the word.

32. D: Answer choice D correctly arranges the ideas to reflect the most effective meaning of the sentence. All other answer choices place the ideas in such a way as to create confusion or incorrect punctuation instead of clarity and correctness.

33. C: In the context, the collective noun *jury* reflects a unit functioning as one, so the word is singular instead of plural. Answer choice C, the singular possessive pronoun *its*, is correct, while answer choice D (the plural *their*) cannot be correct. The word *it's* is the contraction for *it is*. The word *they're* is the contraction for *they are*.

34. A: Answer choice A correctly places the word *compliment* to refer to Amber's positive remark and *complement* to refer to the excellent way that the pieces of furniture work together.

Secret Key #1 - Time is Your Greatest Enemy

Pace Yourself

Wear a watch. At the beginning of the test, check the time (or start a chronometer on your watch to count the minutes), and check the time after every few questions to make sure you are "on schedule."

If you are forced to speed up, do it efficiently. Usually one or more answer choices can be eliminated without too much difficulty. Above all, don't panic. Don't speed up and just begin guessing at random choices. By pacing yourself, and continually monitoring your progress against your watch, you will always know exactly how far ahead or behind you are with your available time. If you find that you are one minute behind on the test, don't skip one question without spending any time on it, just to catch back up. Take 15 fewer seconds on the next four questions, and after four questions you'll have caught back up. Once you catch back up, you can continue working each problem at your normal pace.

Furthermore, don't dwell on the problems that you were rushed on. If a problem was taking up too much time and you made a hurried guess, it must be difficult. The difficult questions are the ones you are most likely to miss anyway, so it isn't a big loss. It is better to end with more time than you need than to run out of time.

Lastly, sometimes it is beneficial to slow down if you are constantly getting ahead of time. You are always more likely to catch a careless mistake by working more slowly than quickly, and among very high-scoring test takers (those who are likely to have lots of time left over), careless errors affect the score more than mastery of material.

Secret Key #2 - Guessing is not Guesswork

You probably know that guessing is a good idea - unlike other standardized tests, there is no penalty for getting a wrong answer. Even if you have no idea about a question, you still have a 20-25% chance of getting it right.

Most test takers do not understand the impact that proper guessing can have on their score. Unless you score extremely high, guessing will significantly contribute to your final score.

Monkeys Take the Test

What most test takers don't realize is that to insure that 20-25% chance, you have to guess randomly. If you put 20 monkeys in a room to take this test, assuming they answered once per question and behaved themselves, on average they would get 20-25% of the questions correct. Put 20 test takers in the room, and the average will be much lower among guessed questions. Why?
    1. The test writers intentionally write deceptive answer choices that "look" right. A test

taker has no idea about a question, so picks the "best looking" answer, which is often wrong. The monkey has no idea what looks good and what doesn't, so will consistently be lucky about 20-25% of the time.

2. Test takers will eliminate answer choices from the guessing pool based on a hunch or intuition. Simple but correct answers often get excluded, leaving a 0% chance of being correct. The monkey has no clue, and often gets lucky with the best choice.

This is why the process of elimination endorsed by most test courses is flawed and detrimental to your performance- test takers don't guess, they make an ignorant stab in the dark that is usually worse than random.

$5 Challenge

Let me introduce one of the most valuable ideas of this course- the $5 challenge:

You only mark your "best guess" if you are willing to bet $5 on it.
You only eliminate choices from guessing if you are willing to bet $5 on it.

Why $5? Five dollars is an amount of money that is small yet not insignificant, and can really add up fast (20 questions could cost you $100). Likewise, each answer choice on one question of the test will have a small impact on your overall score, but it can really add up to a lot of points in the end.

The process of elimination IS valuable. The following shows your chance of guessing it right:

If you eliminate wrong answer choices until only this many remain:	Chance of getting it correct:
1	100%
2	50%
3	33%

However, if you accidentally eliminate the right answer or go on a hunch for an incorrect answer, your chances drop dramatically: to 0%. By guessing among all the answer choices, you are GUARANTEED to have a shot at the right answer.

That's why the $5 test is so valuable- if you give up the advantage and safety of a pure guess, it had better be worth the risk.

What we still haven't covered is how to be sure that whatever guess you make is truly random. Here's the easiest way:

Always pick the first answer choice among those remaining.

Such a technique means that you have decided, **before you see a single test question**, exactly how you are going to guess- and since the order of choices tells you nothing about which one is correct, this guessing technique is perfectly random.

This section is not meant to scare you away from making educated guesses or eliminating choices- you just need to define when a choice is worth eliminating. The $5 test, along with a pre-defined random guessing strategy, is the best way to make sure you reap all of the benefits of guessing.

Secret Key #3 - Practice Smarter, Not Harder

Many test takers delay the test preparation process because they dread the awful amounts of practice time they think necessary to succeed on the test. We have refined an effective method that will take you only a fraction of the time.
There are a number of "obstacles" in your way to succeed. Among these are answering questions, finishing in time, and mastering test-taking strategies. All must be executed on the day of the test at peak performance, or your score will suffer. The test is a mental marathon that has a large impact on your future.

Just like a marathon runner, it is important to work your way up to the full challenge. So first you just worry about questions, and then time, and finally strategy:

Success Strategy

1. Find a good source for practice tests.
2. If you are willing to make a larger time investment, consider using more than one study guide- often the different approaches of multiple authors will help you "get" difficult concepts.
3. Take a practice test with no time constraints, with all study helps "open book." Take your time with questions and focus on applying strategies.
4. Take a practice test with time constraints, with all guides "open book."
5. Take a final practice test with no open material and time limits

If you have time to take more practice tests, just repeat step 5. By gradually exposing yourself to the full rigors of the test environment, you will condition your mind to the stress of test day and maximize your success.

Secret Key #4 - Prepare, Don't Procrastinate

Let me state an obvious fact: if you take the test three times, you will get three different scores. This is due to the way you feel on test day, the level of preparedness you have, and, despite the test writers' claims to the contrary, some tests WILL be easier for you than others.

Since your future depends so much on your score, you should maximize your chances of success. In order to maximize the likelihood of success, you've got to prepare in advance. This means taking practice tests and spending time learning the information and test taking strategies you will need to succeed.

Never take the test as a "practice" test, expecting that you can just take it again if you need to. Feel free to take sample tests on your own, but when you go to take the official test, be prepared, be focused, and do your best the first time!

Secret Key #5 - Test Yourself

Everyone knows that time is money. There is no need to spend too much of your time or too little of your time preparing for the test. You should only spend as much of your precious time preparing as is necessary for you to get the score you need.

Once you have taken a practice test under real conditions of time constraints, then you will know if you are ready for the test or not.
If you have scored extremely high the first time that you take the practice test, then there is not much point in spending countless hours studying. You are already there.

Benchmark your abilities by retaking practice tests and seeing how much you have improved. Once you score high enough to guarantee success, then you are ready.

If you have scored well below where you need, then knuckle down and begin studying in earnest. Check your improvement regularly through the use of practice tests under real conditions. Above all, don't worry, panic, or give up. The key is perseverance!

Then, when you go to take the test, remain confident and remember how well you did on the practice tests. If you can score high enough on a practice test, then you can do the same on the real thing.

General Strategies

The most important thing you can do is to ignore your fears and jump into the test immediately- do not be overwhelmed by any strange-sounding terms. You have to jump into the test like jumping into a pool- all at once is the easiest way.

Make Predictions

As you read and understand the question, try to guess what the answer will be. Remember that several of the answer choices are wrong, and once you begin reading them, your mind will immediately become cluttered with answer choices designed to throw you off. Your mind is typically the most focused immediately after you have read the question and digested its contents. If you can, try to predict what the correct answer will be. You may be surprised at what you can predict.
Quickly scan the choices and see if your prediction is in the listed answer choices. If it is, then you can be quite confident that you have the right answer. It still won't hurt to check the other answer choices, but most of the time, you've got it!

Answer the Question

It may seem obvious to only pick answer choices that answer the question, but the test writers can create some excellent answer choices that are wrong. Don't pick an answer just because it sounds right, or you believe it to be true. It MUST answer the question. Once you've made your selection, always go back and check it against the question and make sure that you didn't misread the question, and the answer choice does answer the question posed.

Benchmark

After you read the first answer choice, decide if you think it sounds correct or not. If it doesn't, move on to the next answer choice. If it does, mentally mark that answer choice. This doesn't mean that you've definitely selected it as your answer choice, it just means that it's the best you've seen thus far. Go ahead and read the next choice. If the next choice is worse than the one you've already selected, keep going to the next answer choice. If the next choice is better than the choice you've already selected, mentally mark the new answer choice as your best guess.

The first answer choice that you select becomes your standard. Every other answer choice must be benchmarked against that standard. That choice is correct until proven otherwise by another answer choice beating it out. Once you've decided that no other answer choice seems as good, do one final check to ensure that your answer choice answers the question posed.

Valid Information

Don't discount any of the information provided in the question. Every piece of information may be necessary to determine the correct answer. None of the information in the question is there to throw you off (while the answer choices will certainly have information to throw you off). If two seemingly unrelated topics are discussed, don't ignore either. You can be confident there is a relationship, or it wouldn't be included in the question, and you are probably going to have to determine what is that relationship to find the answer.

Avoid "Fact Traps"

Don't get distracted by a choice that is factually true. Your search is for the answer that answers the question. Stay focused and don't fall for an answer that is true but incorrect. Always go back to the question and make sure you're choosing an answer that actually answers the question and is not just a true statement. An answer can be factually correct, but it MUST answer the question asked. Additionally, two answers can both be seemingly correct, so be sure to read all of the answer choices, and make sure that you get the one that BEST answers the question.

Milk the Question

Some of the questions may throw you completely off. They might deal with a subject you have not been exposed to, or one that you haven't reviewed in years. While your lack of knowledge about the subject will be a hindrance, the question itself can give you many clues that will help you find the correct answer. Read the question carefully and look for clues. Watch particularly for adjectives and nouns describing difficult terms or words that you don't recognize. Regardless of if you completely understand a word or not, replacing it with a synonym either provided or one you more familiar with may help you to understand what the questions are asking.   Rather than wracking your mind about specific detailed information concerning a difficult term or word, try to use mental substitutes that are easier to understand.

The Trap of Familiarity

Don't just choose a word because you recognize it. On difficult questions, you may not recognize a number of words in the answer choices. The test writers don't put "make-believe" words on the test; so don't think that just because you only recognize all the words in one answer choice means that answer choice must be correct. If you only recognize words in one answer choice, then focus on that one. Is it correct? Try your best to determine if it is correct. If it is, that is great, but if it doesn't, eliminate it. Each word and answer choice you eliminate increases your chances of getting the question correct, even if you then have to guess among the unfamiliar choices.

Eliminate Answers

Eliminate choices as soon as you realize they are wrong. But be careful! Make sure you consider all of the possible answer choices. Just because one appears right, doesn't mean that the next one won't be even better! The test writers will usually put more than one good answer choice for every question, so read all of them. Don't worry if you are stuck between two that seem right. By getting down to just two remaining possible choices, your odds are now 50/50. Rather than wasting too much time, play the odds. You are guessing, but guessing wisely, because you've been able to knock out some of the answer choices that you know are wrong. If you are eliminating choices and realize that the last answer choice you are left with is also obviously wrong, don't panic. Start over and consider each choice again. There may easily be something that you missed the first time and will realize on the second pass.

Tough Questions

If you are stumped on a problem or it appears too hard or too difficult, don't waste time. Move on! Remember though, if you can quickly check for obviously incorrect answer choices, your chances of guessing correctly are greatly improved. Before you completely give up, at least try to knock out a couple of possible answers. Eliminate what you can and then guess at the remaining answer choices before moving on.

Brainstorm

If you get stuck on a difficult question, spend a few seconds quickly brainstorming. Run through the complete list of possible answer choices. Look at each choice and ask yourself, "Could this answer the question satisfactorily?" Go through each answer choice and consider it independently of the other. By systematically going through all possibilities, you may find something that you would otherwise overlook. Remember that when you get stuck, it's important to try to keep moving.

Read Carefully

Understand the problem. Read the question and answer choices carefully. Don't miss the question because you misread the terms. You have plenty of time to read each question thoroughly and make sure you understand what is being asked. Yet a happy medium must be attained, so don't waste too much time. You must read carefully, but efficiently.

Face Value

When in doubt, use common sense. Always accept the situation in the problem at face value. Don't read too much into it. These problems will not require you to make huge leaps of logic. The test writers aren't trying to throw you off with a cheap trick. If you have to go beyond creativity and make a leap of logic in order to have an answer choice answer the question, then you should look at the other answer choices. Don't overcomplicate the problem by creating theoretical relationships or explanations that will warp time or space. These are normal problems rooted in reality. It's just that the applicable relationship or explanation may not be readily apparent and you have to figure things out. Use your common sense to interpret anything that isn't clear.

Prefixes

If you're having trouble with a word in the question or answer choices, try dissecting it. Take advantage of every clue that the word might include. Prefixes and suffixes can be a huge help. Usually they allow you to determine a basic meaning. Pre- means before, post-means after, pro - is positive, de- is negative. From these prefixes and suffixes, you can get an idea of the general meaning of the word and try to put it into context. Beware though of any traps. Just because con is the opposite of pro, doesn't necessarily mean congress is the opposite of progress!

Hedge Phrases

Watch out for critical "hedge" phrases, such as likely, may, can, will often, sometimes, often, almost, mostly, usually, generally, rarely, sometimes. Question writers insert these hedge phrases to cover every possibility. Often an answer choice will be wrong simply because it leaves no room for exception. Avoid answer choices that have definitive words like "exactly," and "always".

Switchback Words

Stay alert for "switchbacks". These are the words and phrases frequently used to alert you to shifts in thought. The most common switchback word is "but". Others include although, however, nevertheless, on the other hand, even though, while, in spite of, despite, regardless of.

New Information

Correct answer choices will rarely have completely new information included. Answer choices typically are straightforward reflections of the material asked about and will directly relate to the question. If a new piece of information is included in an answer choice that doesn't even seem to relate to the topic being asked about, then that answer choice is likely incorrect. All of the information needed to answer the question is usually provided for you, and so you should not have to make guesses that are unsupported or choose answer choices that require unknown information that cannot be reasoned on its own.

Time Management

On technical questions, don't get lost on the technical terms. Don't spend too much time on any one question. If you don't know what a term means, then since you don't have a dictionary, odds are you aren't going to get much further. You should immediately recognize terms as whether or not you know them. If you don't, work with the other clues that you have, the other answer choices and terms provided, but don't waste too much time trying to figure out a difficult term.

Contextual Clues

Look for contextual clues. An answer can be right but not correct. The contextual clues will help you find the answer that is most right and is correct. Understand the context in which a phrase or statement is made. This will help you make important distinctions.

Don't Panic

Panicking will not answer any questions for you. Therefore, it isn't helpful. When you first see the question, if your mind goes blank, take a deep breath. Force yourself to mechanically go through the steps of solving the problem and using the strategies you've learned.

Pace Yourself

Don't get clock fever. It's easy to be overwhelmed when you're looking at a page full of questions, your mind is full of random thoughts and feeling confused, and the clock is ticking down faster than you would like. Calm down and maintain the pace that you have set for yourself. As long as you are on track by monitoring your pace, you are guaranteed to have enough time for yourself. When you get to the last few minutes of the test, it may seem like you won't have enough time left, but if you only have as many questions as you should have left at that point, then you're right on track!

Answer Selection

The best way to pick an answer choice is to eliminate all of those that are wrong, until only one is left and confirm that is the correct answer. Sometimes though, an answer choice may immediately look right. Be careful! Take a second to make sure that the other choices are not equally obvious. Don't make a hasty mistake. There are only two times that you should stop before checking other answers. First is when you are positive that the answer choice you have selected is correct. Second is when time is almost out and you have to make a quick guess!

Check Your Work

Since you will probably not know every term listed and the answer to every question, it is important that you get credit for the ones that you do know. Don't miss any questions through careless mistakes. If at all possible, try to take a second to look back over your answer selection and make sure you've selected the correct answer choice and haven't made a costly careless mistake (such as marking an answer choice that you didn't mean to mark). This quick double check should more than pay for itself in caught mistakes for the time it costs.

Beware of Directly Quoted Answers

Sometimes an answer choice will repeat word for word a portion of the question or reference section. However, beware of such exact duplication – it may be a trap! More than likely, the correct choice will paraphrase or summarize a point, rather than being exactly the same wording.

Slang

Scientific sounding answers are better than slang ones. An answer choice that begins "To compare the outcomes…" is much more likely to be correct than one that begins "Because some people insisted…"

Extreme Statements

Avoid wild answers that throw out highly controversial ideas that are proclaimed as established fact. An answer choice that states the "process should be used in certain situations, if…" is much more likely to be correct than one that states the "process should be discontinued completely." The first is a calm rational statement and doesn't even make a definitive, uncompromising stance, using a hedge word "if" to provide wiggle room, whereas the second choice is a radical idea and far more extreme.

Answer Choice Families

When you have two or more answer choices that are direct opposites or parallels, one of them is usually the correct answer. For instance, if one answer choice states "x increases" and another answer choice states "x decreases" or "y increases," then those two or three answer choices are very similar in construction and fall into the same family of answer choices. A family of answer choices is when two or three answer choices are very similar in construction, and yet often have a directly opposite meaning. Usually the correct answer choice will be in that family of answer choices. The "odd man out" or answer choice that doesn't seem to fit the parallel construction of the other answer choices is more likely to be incorrect.

Special Report: Additional Bonus Material

Due to our efforts to try to keep this book to a manageable length, we've created a link that will give you access to all of your additional bonus material.

Please visit http://www.mometrix.com/bonus948/hobet to access the information.